Cancer and Emotion

Cancer and Emotion
A Practical Guide to Psycho-oncology

Second Edition

JENNIFER BARRACLOUGH*

Consultant in Psychological Medicine
Sir Michael Sobell House
Churchill Hospital
Oxford, UK.

(*Formerly Jennifer Hughes, Department of Psychiatry,
University of Southampton, UK)

JOHN WILEY & SONS
Chichester • New York • Brisbane • Toronto • Singapore

Other Wiley Editorial Offices

John Wiley & Sons, Inc., 605 Third Avenue,
New York, NY 10158-0012, USA

Jacaranda Wiley Ltd, 33 Park Road, Milton,
Queensland 4064, Australia

John Wiley & Sons (Canada) Ltd, 22 Worcester Road,
Rexdale, Ontario M9W 1L1, Canada

John Wiley & Sons (SEA) Pte Ltd, 37 Jalan Pemimpin #05-04,
Block B, Union Industrial Building, Singapore 2057

Library of Congress Cataloging-in-Publication Data

Barraclough, Jennifer.
    Cancer and emotion : a practical guide to psycho-oncology
Jennifer Barraclough
        p.   cm.
    Includes bibliographical references and index.
    ISBN 0 471 93721 5
    1. Cancer—Psychological aspects. I. Title.
    [DNLM: 1. Neoplasms—psychology. 2. Family—psychology.
    3. Psychotherapy. QZ 200 1993]
    RC262.B33 1993
    616.99'4'0019—dc20
DNLM/DLC
For Library of Congress   94–4614
                                                    CIP

British Library Cataloguing in Publication Data

A catalogue record for this book is available from the British Library

ISBN 0 471 93721 5

Typeset in 11/13pt Palatino from author's disks by Production Technology Department,
John Wiley & Sons Ltd, Chichester
Printed and bound in Great Britain by Biddles Ltd, Guildford, Surrey

Contents

Preface
The Scope of Psycho-oncology

What is Psycho-oncology? (Holland 1992)

'Psycho' comes from the Greek word 'psyche' which means the mind or soul.

'Oncology', from the Greek word 'onkos'—a mass—means the study of cancer.

'Psycho-oncology' is concerned with relationships between cancer and the mind. Over the past twenty years it has gained increasing recognition as a medical subspecialty.

'Psychosocial oncology' is a similar term with a broader meaning, reminding us that cancer concerns not just individual patients but their families, friends and workmates, and also the society in which they live.

What is Cancer?

The term 'cancer' covers well over 100 different medical conditions, all involving the abnormal and excessive division of cells. By local tissue invasion, and/or spread to other body parts, cancer threatens the health and life of affected patients.

About one person in three in the Western world will develop cancer during his or her lifetime.

Cancer is sometimes called 'malignant disease'. 'Tumour' and 'growth' are vague alternative terms sometimes used to refer to cancer., though both these words may have other meanings too.

Despite much research, the cause of most forms of cancer is not fully understood. However, a variety of biological factors including genetic makeup, smoking, exposure to certain chemicals, irradiation, excessive sunlight, diet, and virus infection are known to contribute, probably in combination with each other.

Most cancers start off in a localised 'primary site' (the most common ones in Britain being the lung, breast, bowel and prostate) and then, unless treated successfully, spread to produce 'secondaries' or 'metastases' in other parts of the body such as the liver, lungs, bones or brain. As well as being classified by primary site, cancers are subdivided into different 'histological types' on the basis of their cell composition. The most common type is carcinoma; others include sarcoma, lymphoma, and leukaemia.

Both the rate of growth and the pattern of spread vary greatly from case to case.This variation depends partly on the type of cancer concerned, partly on the patient's resistance to it, and partly on the treatment given.

Though cancer retains its traditional reputation as a dread disease, the outlook for cancer patients today is far from hopeless. Some cases can be prevented altogether by avoidance of the risk factors. Early diagnosis, whether by screening programmes or by prompt attention to clinical symptoms, often permits prolonged remission or cure; cure is now possible in about one-third of all cancer cases. Even for patients who cannot be cured, modern methods of symptom control can usually achieve a worthwhile quality of life.

Topics in Psycho-oncology

These include:

• The effects of cancer and its treatment upon the emotional state of patients, their families and the staff who care for them. The emotions which most people associate with cancer are negative ones like anxiety, depression, anger or guilt; but sometimes the disease can have positive effects such as greater appreciation of life or closer personal relationships.

- Ways in which undesirable emotional reactions can be prevented or treated. Do the psychological consequences of cancer depend upon what combination of surgery, chemotherapy and / or radiotherapy are given? Does provision of counselling for newly-diagnosed cancer patients reduce the frequency of emotional disturbance? Are antidepressant drugs helpful to cancer patients who are depressed?
- The possible influence of psychological and social factors upon the development of cancer or its rate of growth. Are people with a passive, compliant type of personality at increased risk of developing cancer—and if so, why? Is the body's resistance to cancer weakened by stressful events such as bereavement? Do patients who put all their energies into fighting their cancer live longer than those with a helpless, hopeless attitude?
- How to introduce research findings into everyday clinical practice. How are diagnostic and treatment services best organised from the psychological point of view? How can oncology staff recognise the emotionally distressed patient in busy wards and clinics? Who should provide psychosocial care? How many patients would benefit from specialised counselling—and how many actually want it?

A great deal of the work done in psycho-oncology has been focused on breast cancer. The reasons for this are not difficult to understand; breast cancer is common (and becoming more so), afflicts high numbers of young articulate women who are well-motivated to take part in psychosocial inquiries, and carries obvious threats to body image and sexuality as well as to physical health and survival. Breast cancer is certainly a very important condition but has perhaps received more than its fair share of attention, from the psychosocial aspect, compared with other forms of the disease. Bowel cancer, for example, may well have even more distressing psychosocial and psychosexual effects than breast cancer does, yet research studies are far fewer and less well publicised.

Whereas some topics in psycho-oncology are specific to a particular form of cancer, others have a more general application. Site-specific issues (such as reactions to mastectomy or colostomy) are of most relevance for localised early cancers, whereas general issues (such as psychological adjustment to dying) predominate for patients with advanced cancer. Many of the general issues are also relevant to other chronic life-threatening physical illnesses besides cancer: for example heart disease, degenerative neurological conditions, and AIDS.

Factors Shaping Response

A patient's psychological response to cancer depends on many different factors:

- Physical prognosis, as understood by the patient. Some cancers can be permanently cured, some are almost certain to be fatal, and many others lie somewhere in between. Prognosis can seldom be accurately predicted for the individual case, but guidelines can be given depending on what type of cancer is involved, and its stage of advancement when diagnosed.
- Age, sex and social group of the patient. The psychosocial issues for a retired male manual worker who is suffering from lung cancer, for example, will probably be rather different from those affecting a young professional woman with breast cancer.
- Cause of the disease. Is there any reason for patients to blame themselves (smokers who develop lung cancer) or other people (asbestos workers who develop mesothelioma)—or, as for so many forms of cancer, is the patient faced with the unanswerable question 'why me?'?
- Symptoms of the disease. Is there obvious bodily disfigurement, as with tumours of the head and neck, or an invisible internal growth such as cancer of the pancreas causing constant pain and sapping of strength?
- Direct effects of the disease and its treatment on brain function, for example cerebral metastases, biochemical disturbances, drugs with an effect on mood. *chemo - brain*
- Psychological effects of the treatment given: a mutilating operation (mastectomy, colostomy), nausea, vomiting and hair loss (with some forms of radiotherapy and chemotherapy), prolonged interference with work and social life through repeated hospital attendance.
- Stigma, although this is now much less than was once the case. Ten or twenty years ago, so much secrecy surrounded the

subject of cancer that it was common medical practice to conceal this diagnosis from the patient. Nowadays the diagnosis is almost always disclosed, and the word 'cancer' is openly spoken in some social circles though not all.

- The patient's relationship with doctors and nurses. This may be permanently influenced by the way that news of the diagnosis was conveyed at the beginning.
- Characteristics of the patient as a person: past life experience, personality, family relationships, religious beliefs, and current social circumstances.

About this Book

My aim has been to write an introductory overview in non-technical language. The emphasis throughout is a practical one, concerned largely with the psychosocial impact of cancer and its treatment upon patients, families and staff, and the mangement of clinical problems arising from this. It deals only with cancer in adults; childhood cancer is an equally important subject but I am not qualified to write about it.

I hope the book will contain material of interest and value to the following groups:

- Nurses, doctors and other staff who provide physical care for cancer patients in radiotherapy, oncology, and other medical and surgical units in general hospitals.
- Staff of palliative care units (hospices).
- Mental health professionals carrying out consultation–liaison work in cancer treatment settings.
- Members of primary health care teams, most of whom will be looking after a number of patients with cancer at any one time.
- Interested members of the general public, who sometimes gain a distorted picture from presentations in the popular media.
- Cancer patients themselves, their families and friends.

My main audience will probably be nurses and doctors looking after cancer patients in hospital. Any items of direct advice to the reader are, therefore, addressed towards this group.

The book is divided into seven parts, with suggestions for further reading given at the end of each. Many of these are chapters from the large American textbook which is the standard reference work in this field: *Handbook of Psychooncology*, edited by JC Holland and JH Rowland, published in 1989 by Oxford University Press. Review articles from other sources are also included.

The patients I have known over the years have been a major source of inspiration to me in writing this book, and I would like to express my thanks to them. Most of the chapters include clinical case histories. All these are based on real patients, but names and identifying details have been changed to preserve confidentiality, and sometimes two cases have been rolled into one. The exception is 'Me: Why Me?' written by Hilary Scott, in her own words under her own name, and reproduced in a slightly abridged version by kind permission of her husband Roy. I also wish to thank the many colleagues at Sir Michael Sobell House who, whether through informal discussion or specific comments on the manuscript, have helped me with this project.

FURTHER READING

Holland JC (1992) Psychooncology: overview, obstacles and opportunities. *Psycho-oncology 1* 1–13

"Me: Why Me?"—One Patient's Story

There was no premonition that this day would dramatically change the rest of my life. I found a walnut-sized lump in my left breast, and so began the course of events which continue, after six years, to test my strength and courage beyond what I believed possible.

"You have a growth," pronounced the surgeon, bending over me as I lay on the paper-covered hospital examining table. It seemed an obvious remark. My question sounded casual "Do you mean a malignant growth?" I don't know how I expected him to reply, but I didn't think he would be so sure when he said that in his opinion it was malignant.

(Somewhere, in the back of my mind, though, the diagnosis seemed inevitable. I had often felt that cancer would be my fate; my mother had died of it in her late 40s.)

So this is what it feels like to be told you have cancer. Shock, numbness, fear, unreality—this can't actually be happening to me.

The actual word cancer had been carefully avoided—something I have found over the years to be a very common omission. So much so, that when my daughter and I recently saw a genetic counsellor and every other word he said was cancer, or breast cancer, we got the giggles, as it has become a standing joke to talk of oncology, disease, tumour, but not the dreaded word!

A friend had told me the previous day that nine out of ten lumps are benign, but I thought, cynically at the time, someone has to be the unlucky one. And now it appeared to be me. The surgeon explained to me and my husband that he planned a segmental

continued

continued

mastectomy, to remove a wedge of my left breast, and that the operation would be followed by a course of radiotherapy, as a safety measure, to destroy any cancer cells left behind.

It was January 1986, and he advised taking until Easter off from my job as a playgroup supervisor. Suddenly I was out of control of my life; cancer had invaded my body and terror was fast invading my mind.

And so it all began; my long battle with cancer. But for years I had been fighting another battle against the insidious depression, anxiety and panic which frequently engulfed me. Many, many times all I wanted to do was to give up on everything, shrink into oblivion and find peace—death seemed the only way to be free. And now I had come face to face with death. The experience of cancer has changed my life.

When I began to read all I could about breast cancer, in early 1986, I discovered that I appeared to fit almost too perfectly into the typical "cancer personality". I had suffered from anxiety and depression since the age of eleven. I had been hospitalised on numerous occasions, seen various psychiatrists, taken literally hundreds of antidepressants and tranquillisers, all in an attempt to put to flight the huge black bird which so often seemed to be perching on my shoulder, causing total despair and several suicide attempts. I was completely at odds with the world. I found relationships very difficult as I was constantly afraid of rejection; I suffered severe panic attacks, which for years prevented me from going out and about and leading a normal life. Life was a continual struggle: I felt totally inadequate and unsatisfied with everything. So, when I was diagnosed as having breast cancer, this is how I was, unhappy, anxious, insecure.

In January 1986, aged 38, when I discovered my breast cancer I was working at playgroup several sessions a week. I was getting out and about, teaching in Sunday school and generally leading a more normal life. But I was still unhappy with myself and my inability to control my emotions. A shopping trip to Oxford was still an ordeal, due to panic attacks.

The planned operation on my breast went ahead—I amazed myself at how well I managed to get through it all, but I came home feeling pleased with myself because I had maintained my self-control. My faith in God was very real at this time; I felt able to trust him as never before and I was able to take courage from this and from the loving support of family and friends.

continued

continued

The surgeon who had operated on my breast had misled me into thinking that the cancer hadn't spread when, in fact, at my first appointment with the radiotherapy consultant I was told that the treatment would have to be very aggressive as the cancer involved my lymph nodes.

Chemotherapy was discussed and I went home "to think about it". How can one think about a course of action without relevant information? I needed to be fairly well informed before I could ask questions. I decided that chemotherapy seemed to offer a reasonable chance of destroying any cancer cells which may be lurking around, and began the recommended course. This turned out to be worse than I had anticipated; I found the nausea and vomiting very distressing and I had an allergic reaction to the anti-sickness drugs.

On the fourth course of treatment my husband and I were put in a side room, after the preliminary blood tests, and left waiting for an hour. The doctor then appeared with the prepared drugs and syringes. I began to cry, and he told me not to go ahead if I didn't feel like it—of course I didn't; who would? He told us that he would refrigerate the drugs and we could go away for an hour or so to decide what I wanted to do.

How could we decide what was best: all I knew was that I had reached the end of my endurance that day and I couldn't face the treatment. I was told, on my return, that if I didn't have the injections that day I may as well give up altogether. And that is what I did. But advice and counselling were non-existent.

The radiotherapy went ahead as planned. I found it very difficult: lying trapped under huge machines, for four minutes at a time, was very claustrophobic—just the kind of situation which filled me with terror. But I developed a coping strategy, learning to relax by singing in my head, a favourite song being "Be still and know that I am God". I emerged from the radiotherapy badly burned. It was impossible to wear any clothes for several days as they stuck to the burns.

I remember a Sunday school outing to Moreton-in-the-Marsh. As I didn't feel well enough to attempt the train journey with fifty or sixty children, my husband Roy took me in the car and despite the painful burns and generally feeling unwell we had a lovely afternoon, surrounded by children and friends and sharing a picnic tea.

At this stage in the proceedings—July 1986—I went to Bristol Cancer Help Centre. I had read *A Gentle Way With Cancer* and

continued

continued

had watched the television programmes about the centre. Their approach was new and refreshing. No one even asked to see my breast; at the hospital that seemed to be their only area of interest. I was treated as a person, my dis-ease was considered.

The treatment I had received was excellent, and I was grateful that we were fortunate enough to live near such a good hospital, but I felt that I was treated as a carcinoma left breast and the rest of me was ignored. To me, it was a very personal thing, my cancer, a threat to my life, my courage, my faith in God, my entire existence.

I desperately needed to feel that I could still maintain some measure of control over my life and my destiny and come to terms with my illness and the way it affected me. My way of dealing with this was to meet it face on, and I needed to talk about it. My husband was very supportive, taking me to and from clinics, and looking after me through the side-effects of the treatment.

But his method of coping was the opposite to mine, being that if it wasn't thought or talked about it might actually go away.

The day we spent together at Bristol was a revelation to me. I came away feeling positive about my illness and that I was able to take an active part in helping myself find wholeness. Apart from the cancer I was a very emotionally wounded and battered person.

I began to practise relaxation and meditation, and read the Simonton book *Getting Well Again*. I found some of the recommendations about diet and supplements a bit way out, but we were largely vegetarian already, and I did cut out tea and coffee. So I took what I found helpful from Bristol.

Gradually, normal life resumed, and in September 1986 I was able to return to work at playgroup, eight months after I had left.

But about six months after all the treatment ended the full impact of what had happened seemed to hit me—I had coped far better than I believed possible at the time, now I went to pieces. In retrospect this was a very "normal" reaction. I spent a couple of weeks in a psychiatric hospital, and it was at this time that I first met a psychiatrist who has become a kind and trusted friend over the years. He always sees me and Roy together, and for the first time I began to feel a lessening of the guilt and blame attached to always being labelled "ill", if not physically, then mentally.

The following summer we went as a family, and accompanied by my father, to Orkney, to visit my younger brother and his family who have settled there. This trip presented me with a real challenge: train, boat and bus journeys—but I managed

continued

continued

it, and the wonderful holiday was crowned with a sense of achievement.

My hospital checkups had gradually lengthened to every six months and I was feeling very well and optimistic when in June 1988 I found a small lump in my right breast. The whole process began again. It was a tremendous blow to my confidence that after over two years the cancer had returned, and indeed to come to the realisation that all the time it had been silently lurking within my body.

I went ahead and had a lumpectomy, and returned to Bristol a week after the operation. Again I came determined to get the better of the disease, using whatever means I could, orthodox medicine, alternative medicine and Christian healing. I felt much more positive about myself as a person and my ability to cope with my illness.

The course of radiotherapy was not as intensive as the first time, as my lymph nodes were not involved. I employed much the same methods of coping, including visualisation learnt at Bristol and through Carl Simonton's book *Getting Well Again*. By October I was back at work, planning Christmas parties and nativity plays as usual.

The next year or so passed reasonably smoothly. My son Matthew left home in June 1989 to live and work in Oxford. One, for me, momentous occasion worth recording was that at the Christmas candlelight service on Christmas Eve 1989 I walked to the lectern in front of a packed church and read the lesson—Luke chapter 2 "And there were at that time, shepherds abiding in the fields".

The tremendous thing about it was that less than a year before I couldn't even sit in church without feelings of panic. The feeling of achievement was tremendous. Half the congregation were children, and from my work at playgroup I knew almost every child between twelve and three.

My work at playgroup continued and I became involved with setting up a new group of Rainbow Guides (5–7 year olds; pre-Brownies).

Depression was still troublesome, but on the whole life was much more stable. I loved my work with children. Roy and I still saw Pepé the psychiatrist every couple of months or so.

In March 1990 I had what I assumed to be an ear infection, but although I went to the GP complaining of pain there was no

continued

continued

infection. Then the pain seemed to be in my jaw and I saw my dentist who told me it was nothing to worry about—as did my GP when I visited him again, even though by now the pain was unrelenting, like toothache and earache together, and my face was swollen.

By July there was no improvement and my doctor suggested ultrasound treatment. At the end of July I went to camp with the Guides, and I noticed that my right side felt stiff and painful sometimes, and by the end of the week my neck was also very stiff. But it seemed reasonable to suppose this could be the result of camping.

At a further visit to the doctor I was told to return in a week if my neck had not improved. Meanwhile the ultrasound treatment to my jaw continued, and when I mentioned my now ever increasing catalogue of aches and pains to the physiotherapist, she wrote to my doctor. As a result of this, he carried out some blood tests which, he said, showed that I had arthritis. I was reassured by this, because I knew that breast cancer readily metastasises in bone, and I had been worried.

I voiced my concern to my GP and suggested a bone scan. There was a definite lump on my jaw, as well as pain in my ribs, neck and legs. I felt unwell and had lost $1\frac{1}{2}$ stones in weight. By this time it was August and we were due to visit our son in Canada. I was having difficulty walking, my neck was extremely painful, it was impossible to move my head a fraction of an inch without intense pain, and I spent some nights sitting propped up on the sofa, unable to sleep.

So I went again to my doctor who arranged for me to see an arthritis specialist. The specialist immediately suggested a bone scan, and I was able to arrange this rapidly through a friend who is a radiographer. After an exhausting day of scans and X-rays I had to visit my GP yet again for the results. My suspicions were confirmed—I had metastases in my ribs, jaw and pelvis. Apparently nothing had shown up in my jaw in the scan, but I pointed out the swelling to the radiographer who X-rayed it.

My neck was increasingly painful, and a further X-ray revealed a critical situation: disease had almost destroyed the odontoid peg. I was advised to cancel my holiday and have since learned from one of the people who influenced this decision that she was torn between advising me to go and risk breaking my neck, or to stay and possibly never see my son again.

continued

continued

My husband and daughter went to Canada as planned and I stayed and had radiotherapy on my neck, jaw and pubic bone. Within six weeks I had changed from a busy, active person, into a disabled one in a wheelchair, with my neck in a hard collar. But not only that, I had changed into a dying person.

I realised that this time the cancer was terminal, and this knowledge brought with it many conflicting emotions. One of the first things I felt was grief for my husband and children, and for the grandchildren I may never see. I was determined that if I had to die I would live life to the full until I died. I tried to find some purpose in my suffering. I prayed for healing.

I had to tell Matthew the state of affairs by telephone—a heartbreaking task. I wanted both children to know and understand what was happening and they have always been fully informed.

Roy and I spent a few days in the Yorkshire Dales. I wasn't very mobile, and encased in a hard collar, but managed a walk around Fountains Abbey, and the cream cakes from Betty's in Harrogate were a real treat.

Matthew came home in December and we had a lovely family Christmas, a poignant time, would it be our last? I had been forced to give up my job at playgroup and I found sitting in on the Christmas party very sad. I organised the costumes for the Sunday school nativity play as usual, but found it almost impossible to watch the children's performance. I felt so sad and unsure of my future.

The pain in my neck improved enormously although I still wore a hard collar day and night. I was put on tamoxifen with no real effect, and had more palliative radiation to a rib which had fractured. Radiotherapy to my lower back and left hip became necessary in February, to help the pain.

In mid-March, Roy and I went to Florence and to Venice. Although walking was painful, I managed a full programme of sightseeing with my wheelchair. And at long last I had conquered my fear of flying. I wouldn't go so far as to say that I actually enjoyed it, but I did it, and the sight of the clouds beneath us illuminated by sunshine was incredible and unforgettable.

In April my left hip fractured, and one Monday afternoon I found myself in Casualty. The consultant discussed his plan to pin the bone the following morning, but I insisted that I wanted to attend a wedding on the coming Thursday. The doctors, frankly,

continued

continued

didn't seem too keen on letting me go home with a fractured neck of femur, but with encouragement from one of the nurses to stick up for what I wanted, I arranged to be re-admitted on the Friday, the day after the wedding.

I should explain that this was no ordinary wedding. My friend was marrying for the second time and Roy and I had been asked to be witnesses—no one else knew about it. We had a very special day, and I duly presented myself at the hospital on the Friday.

The surgeon had decided that my hip was too badly diseased to pin, and so I underwent a hip replacement under an epidural as my neck and jaw were still unstable. My recovery was quick, and on the whole the week's stay in hospital uneventful.

One incident does, however, stand out. I suffered from headaches as a result of the epidural, and about three days after the operation a blood patch was done. Some blood was drawn, via a cannula, and injected into my spine, the idea being that the blood would clot and seal the small hole where fluid was leaking. This went well, and the cannula was left in place as it had been discovered that I needed a blood transfusion.

A young woman doctor came with the blood, but it would not flow through the cannula in my right arm. So she proceeded to make two attempts on my left arm, with complete and total disregard for me. I was, by this time, near to the end of my endurance. One kind word, or even an acknowledgement that attached to that arm was a person, would have made so much difference to me.

Instead I sat on the bed with tears silently streaming down my face, more from lack of simple caring than pain. A word of encouragement, a touch or a smile, can make so much difference to the situation. Patients are people, and what is more we are frequently frightened and feeling extremely vulnerable.

Whilst having radiation treatment planned to my hip, I was lying on a table. Although the consultant surgeon came to look at the X-rays, he didn't even look my way, let alone acknowledge my presence. I wish I had the courage to sit up and say "Good morning, by the way attached to this hip is a living, rather insecure person". Just a couple of words would have made so much difference.

Medical students should be taught much more about patients as people. Before my second breast operation I was asked if I minded students coming in with the consultant. I readily agreed, and all went well. But after the physical examination and chat the

continued

continued

consultant and ten students went just outside the door and proceeded to discuss my case within my hearing and that of my two room-mates who had no idea why I was there until then.

Dignity is very important, too. I had an eight minute radiotherapy treatment to my pubic bone, and was told by the radiographers not to take my underwear off, just to slip it down. But did they not consider what it feels like to be lying on the treatment table for eight minutes with my knickers round my knees? I felt thoroughly miserable and humiliated: a blanket over my underwear and knees would have meant so much.

Summer 1991 was spent doing all sorts of things which I had thought I would never again be able to manage. We spent two weekends at a friend's caravan in Wales and only six weeks after the hip replacement I climbed up and down to Welsh beaches and walked on the sand. We also spent two weekends in Norfolk, and on one occasion I walked about two miles over tidal marshes to an island, and returned after a picnic lunch, in a small ferry. I climbed in at one end, and walked down a gangplank at the other!

A particular joy has been my ability to walk again in Wychwood forest, a place which I love, and I had thought would not be accessible again. Being able to go on these walks was taken for granted a couple of years ago: this summer they meant so much more because I had thought I would never do them again. My life has been enriched in so many ways through the experience of cancer.

It is now November 1991. Having cancer has been a very educational process for me, and I have met so much love and help along the way. I still sometimes think, why me? The age old question of why we have to suffer has not been fully answered, but I do know now that suffering can be used to bring about a greater trust and confidence in God, and also in oneself. I now feel very secure in the knowledge that God is very close to me in my pain.

So why choose me to endure this? I'm not tough enough, I haven't the strength and courage. In fact, I'm an extremely bad candidate with my long history of anxiety and depression. I am not special, I am just an ordinary person having to deal with cancer. But if I can do it, then so can anyone.

Why was I selected to take on this task? I believe that it was to lead me to wholeness and healing and that I am discovering these gifts through my suffering. I have grown enormously,

continued

continued

emotionally and spiritually. I needed to come to terms with my illness, and in doing that I am being freed to find healing in and through it.

I have learned to trust God, and other people, and to ask for help. I have found a stronger faith, and I am certain that wherever I am, in pain, terror, depression, God is always there beside me. My courage has increased enormously with this knowledge.

In a strange way having cancer has given me a purpose in life which was lacking before. It is certainly a challenge—just to get up each day and live with it, but much more to try to bring something positive out of the experience. With my increasing confidence in God my old angers and bitterness have largely vanished. I have found so much love and support from family, friends, doctors and nurses, and I have become much more secure and able to accept love and help without the old fear of rejection. And, I think, more able to give something back to other people.

Healing isn't necessarily physical healing, but wholeness, and a tremendous amount of healing has taken place in me. I have discovered various allies along the way—relaxation, meditation, yoga, massage, aromatherapy.

I am thankful for the people I have met—friends who have encouraged me enormously and supported me with cards, letters, phone calls, prayers, love and their confidence in me. For the doctors I have met, and the nurses who have looked after me, and for the nurses and volunteers at Sir Michael Sobell House, our local hospice. For fellow patients, for their friendship, courage and humour. For a chance meeting with a priest in Walsingham, and the relationship which has developed, and for the friendship of Pepé. And for the concern of so many people, too numerous to mention.

There is still an enormous stigma attached to cancer, but I think that it is most important to let people know that the disease is not an immediate death sentence. I am alive and reasonably well, I lead a very full life. I am a survivor and so are thousands of others. We should let people know.

Our illness may be terminal—life is terminal! A patient support group has been set up at Sir Michael Sobell House and this is an encouraging development. We have been asked to video a group session for teaching purposes. I was asked a few weeks ago if I would allow a medical student to interview me about my feelings. So things are changing.

continued

continued

I am, at the moment, deciding whether to undergo some palliative radiotherapy to my pelvis. This time I feel that I am firmly in control. I have learnt to become more assertive and to fit my treatment into my life rather than having to fit my life around my treatment.

Undergoing a bone scan recently I asked if I could use my Walkman. The technician said, "No one ever asked before". So I was able to listen to Pavarotti and recall, while having my scan, a wet but very memorable day spent in Hyde Park. What a difference from lying alone and afraid looking at the ceiling!

As for the future—who knows—there is so much to look forward to. Maybe another trip to Italy in the Spring? A great joy, being godmother to my friend's baby daughter in January, and a party in July to celebrate several special family birthdays.

I only visited Bristol Cancer Help Centre twice, but I always feel a sense of caring and peace when I go through the front door. Although I haven't been an avid follower of their philosophy, a lot of their suggestions have helped me in the journey I am undertaking, and I feel a lasting gratitude to them for helping me to see my disease and my life differently.

Sometimes I still feel angry. I often feel vulnerable, but I rarely feel alone. People's kindness and generosity continue to help me. Throughout it all I have retained a sense of humour. I am a different person, I have changed, and it seems sad that the change has had to come about with the onset of a life-threatening illness, but I am thankful that the change has taken place.

I have wonderful friends. I couldn't manage without their support and their confidence in my ability to continue to be me; somewhat scarred by my experiences but nevertheless a whole person. I like to be treated as I always was, but for people not to ignore what is happening to me, because cancer has become a part of my life whether I like it or not.

Hilary Scott, 28 June 1947–10 March 1992

©1993, Executors of Hilary Scott, reproduced with permission in abridged form.

1
The Impact of Diagnosis and Treatment

The psychological impact of learning a diagnosis of cancer depends to some extent on the way the disease presents. Diagnosis should be a reasonably straightforward process for those patients who have noticed early symptoms of a classical kind and promptly sought medical advice. It may be a more confused and long-drawn-out affair when the case is medically complex, or the doctor has failed to investigate it properly, or the patient has concealed the symptoms for some time. At the other extreme, diagnosis can come as a sudden bolt from the blue when cancer is discovered unexpectedly in an apparently healthy person. Various scenarios are considered below.

Diagnosis is usually followed by treatment. Psychological aspects of anticancer treatment in general will be discussed, then the three main types—surgery, chemotherapy, and radiotherapy—considered in turn. A note on complementary (alternative) therapies is also included.

THE DIAGNOSTIC PROCESS

Every patient is different—but certain common patterns occur. A typical sequence of events surrounding the diagnosis of cancer, and psychological reactions to these, would be as follows.

The clinical story begins when a person develops some troublesome or worrying physical symptom and consults the family doctor. Suspicion of cancer may or may not already exist in the mind of doctor and/or patient at this time. A lump in the breast or bleeding from bladder or bowel will probably arouse immediate fears, whereas vaguer symptoms like loss of weight or repeated chest infections may not. Appreciation that something may be seriously wrong gradually increases, perhaps as a result of physical examination, or blood tests or X-rays, or the symptoms getting worse. Hospital referral will probably be arranged, and more specialised tests carried out, before a definite diagnosis can be made and treatment options discussed.

This process may take days, weeks or months, but is usually sufficiently gradual for the possibility of cancer to have been planted in the patient's mind, and considered either inwardly or in discussion with others, before it is confirmed. Many patients find this period of uncertainty so stressful that receiving a definite diagnosis of cancer actually comes as a relief to them. Administrative delays in health service settings should be kept to a minimum not just because prompt treatment is medically desirable, but because waiting even a few days for the result of a biopsy or an X-ray can provoke intense anxiety.

The way the diagnosis is explained to the patient may have a major and lasting effect on his or her adjustment to it; practical guidance about conducting a 'bad news consultation' will be given later in the book.

Coming to terms with cancer, once this has been confirmed, often involves a progression through various emotional stages:

1. Shock, numbness or disbelief on first learning the truth; the bad news seems too much to 'take in'. This may be called the stage of denial and usually lasts no more than a few days.
2. Acute distress as the full reality dawns: anxiety, anger, bargaining and protest, often lasting several weeks.
3. Depression and despair, which may also last several weeks.
4. Gradual adjustment and acceptance, often taking several months.

This well-known model, based on Elizabeth Kubler-Ross's work with terminally ill patients, has also proved a most useful framework for understanding the adjustment to an initial cancer diagnosis. A similar sequence is found after diagnosis of other serious illnesses, after bereavement, and indeed after many other kinds of 'life events' which involve an important loss, for example being made redundant or being deserted by one's partner. The model should not be applied too rigidly, because wide variations from the classic sequence are frequently found and are not necessarily undesirable. Some patients demonstrate calm acceptance (Stage 4) from the start; some undergo belated adjustment reactions (Stages 2 and 3) well after the initial diagnosis; others remain fixed in denial (Stage 1), or else revert back to this stage if and when their physical condition deteriorates.

Variations to the pattern of disease presentation described above are frequent. Some patients are diagnosed suddenly and unexpectedly, for example if they go into hospital for an apparently minor condition and are found to have evidence of cancer on physical examination, on X-ray, or during the course of a surgical operation for something else. Two important variations will be discussed in more detail: diagnosis by screening, and diagnostic delay.

SCREENING (Wardle and Pope 1992)

Screening programmes involve testing defined populations for the presence of specified cancers, precancerous conditions and risk factors for cancer. Two separate national screening programmes currently operate for women of certain age-bands in the UK: one for breast cancer (mammography), one for cancer of the cervix (cervical smears).

The aim of screening programmes is to improve cancer prognosis through early diagnosis and treatment. How far they actually succeed in this aim can only be established by largescale research studies. There is evidence that breast cancer screening can reduce breast cancer mortality by about 25% (though probably only for women over 50 years of age). Knowledge regarding the value of screening for other common cancers, such as those of the prostate, ovary and bowel, is not yet available. Any benefits of screening programmes must be balanced against their demands on health service resources, and possible adverse effects whether physical or psychological. The psychological costs will be briefly considered in relation to various groups:

- *People who refuse screening* (about 20%) are often just the ones who would benefit most, because many of them come from the same socially deprived sections of the population which are at greatest risk of cancer and/or tend to present their symptoms late. Some of those who refuse have undoubtedly been distressed or frightened by the invitation letter, perhaps misinterpreting it to mean that that they are already suffering from cancer. It is impossible to know how frequent or severe such extreme reactions are, because badly affected people will also refuse any kind of research inquiry.
- *Healthy people whose screening tests yield normal results* form the largest group. Followup studies have not demonstrated any major lasting psychological effects in such people, though many report transient anxiety around the actual screening procedure, and subtle longterm changes may occur. Screened people become more aware of their risk of developing cancer; a desirable change if it leads to a healthier lifestyle or prompter reporting of suspicious symptoms in the future, but not so desirable if accompanied by persistent mild anxiety or hypochondriasis which impairs their enjoyment of life. Many people are pleased to receive a normal test result but it is important to make sure they are not lulled into false security, because a normal test on one occasion does not guarantee freedom from cancer in future.
- *Those who develop symptoms of cancer shortly after a normal screening test* may either be suffering from a very fast-growing form of cancer, or may for a variety of reasons have been given a 'false negative' result. Patients in this situation may be understandably upset that the screening test has failed them—especially if, because of the reassurance given, further tests have been delayed.
- *Those found to have an abnormality of uncertain significance:* some of the very early cancers, or precancerous conditions, which can be detected by screening might never have given rise to clinical disease during the person's lifetime. However, because there is no way of predicting which cases of this kind will progress and

which will not, it is usual practice to offer treatment and/or frequent followup to all those in whom a precancerous abnormality is found. Many people find it hard to understand the concept of precancerous conditions. A clear and sympathetic explanation may well minimise psychological distress for this group.

- *'False positives'*: not all suspicious screening test results turn out to be significant after fuller investigation. Some of those who receive an 'all-clear' after an initial false alarm will be left with lasting anxiety or anger, feeling they have endured great psychological trauma for no good reason. The length of time taken to resolve the issue is important here. Anyone found to have abnormal smears or mammograms should be followed up as quickly as possible, not left in suspense.

- *Those found to have invasive cancer* may be considered fortunate if the early diagnosis of their disease permits successful treatment. However, the diagnosis may come as an even greater shock than when it is made in the usual way after clinical symptoms have developed. (In contrast to tests for HIV disease, screening tests for cancer are not routinely preceded by detailed counselling about what the implications of a positive result might be.) For an unfortunate minority of patients, the screening diagnosis brings little or no advantage, either because the cancer is already advanced when found or because it continues to advance despite treatment. Such patients might have been better off remaining in ignorance for a longer period.

Scientific knowledge about the molecular genetics of cancer is increasing rapidly at the present time. This will permit more sophisticated screening regarding an individual's risk of developing specified forms of cancer within his or her lifetime. Such new techniques are likely to raise complicated issues about the ethics of screening, whether within affected families or for the population as a whole.

Potential negative aspects of cancer screening have been highlighted here, but it must be emphasised that these apply to a minority of subjects only and that, on present evidence, screening for cancers of both breast and cervix is to be encouraged because it does save lives.

DELAY (Holland 1989a)

Delay in the diagnosis of cancer is undesirable because, as a general rule, later diagnosis means less successful treatment.

Some people seek medical advice immediately if they notice a symptom which might signify cancer. Others wait a few days or weeks to think over the situation, probably hoping that meantime the symptom may go away; or deliberately put off taking any action until, for example, a booked holiday or a child's wedding has taken place.

While the sooner treatment is started the better, delays of a few weeks probably make little difference to the final outcome in most cases. Delay lasting months rather than weeks is more serious. Research studies about delay often focus on patients in whom the interval from first symptom to diagnosis is more than three to six months.

Either patient or doctor may be responsible for delay.

Patient delay may be linked to the following factors:

- *Ignorance:* some patients, especially the elderly or the poorly educated, do not realise the potential significance of certain symptoms. For example, although almost all women know that a lump in the breast should be taken seriously, some do not appreciate that other symptoms such as nipple discharge or inversion may also signify cancer. Others believe that cancer is always fatal so there is no point in seeking treatment.
- *Anxiety:* some patients are so terrified of cancer they dare not go to the doctor. Many of these are badly informed about modern treatments. Old wives' tales remembered from long ago, or their own secret fantasies, paint an unduly black mental picture.
- *Denial:* these patients are also assumed, at one level, to be terrified of cancer but are able to block out this anxiety from conscious awareness. They claim they did not notice any symptoms, or thought their symptoms were unimportant, and appear quite unconcerned about what is wrong.
- *Conscious choice:* as in the case of the elderly woman who deliberately concealed her breast tumour for three years because she wanted to stay at home to nurse her sick husband.

She was eventually driven to seek medical help by severe backache due to bony metastases.

- *Embarrassment:* cancers of the bowel, bladder, and sexual organs give rise to symptoms which some patients are reluctant to discuss. Asian women immigrants to the UK form one particular group who, because of modesty, may fail to seek advice about early symptoms of breast or genital cancers.
- *Psychiatric disorder:* cancer in patients suffering from such conditions as chronic schizophrenia, mental handicap or Alzheimer's disease may go undetected for a long time unless regular medical examinations are carried out.

Doctor delay, in which a general practitioner (GP) or hospital specialist fails to make the correct diagnosis when the patient first presents, ranges from the unavoidable to the negligent.

Cherry, aged 24, consulted her general practitioner (GP) because of colicky abdominal pains and diarrhoea. Physical examination showed nothing abnormal and, knowing that Cherry was under some stress both at work and at home at the time, the doctor diagnosed an anxiety state and prescribed a course of diazepam. A few months later, when Cherry's diarrhoea had got worse and she was losing weight, the same GP arranged some physical investigations which revealed cancer of the bowel. This doctor was much troubled with self-reproach. However, Cherry herself said he could not have been expected to make the right diagnosis at first.

Because GPs cannot be expected to carry out extensive tests on every young, healthy-looking patient who presents with a common and non-specific symptom, it is inevitable that cases like this are sometimes missed. Delays may also arise if the cancer presents with atypical symptoms, when the results of tests are inconclusive or when the patient has other medical pathology which complicates the diagnosis. In such situations, again, delay is unfortunate but excusable.

In other cases the doctor has no excuse. Another young woman presented with vaginal bleeding between periods: the doctor who prescribed the contraceptive pill without doing a vaginal examination was guilty of negligence. When that patient was seen by a different doctor six months later, she was found to have an advanced carcinoma of the cervix.

Patients are often angry with the doctor whom they hold responsible for diagnostic delay. This feeling may be perfectly justified, or it may reflect their own imperfect understanding of a complex clinical situation, or their need to find some target for their anger about the cancer itself. Assessing the true rights and wrongs of the case may be impossible.

Better education for both doctors and patients would help prevent delay.

PRINCIPLES OF ANTICANCER TREATMENT

Three main kinds of treatment—surgery, chemotherapy (including cytotoxic drugs and hormones), and radiotherapy—are used alone or in combination for treating cancer. As a general rule, surgery and radiotherapy are given for cancers localised to certain parts of the body whereas chemotherapy is appropriate for widespread disease.

These three modalities are sometimes called 'specific' or 'active' treatments, because they are designed to eliminate the cancer completely or at least slow down its progression. This distinguishes them from 'symptomatic' treatments such as pain-reducing drugs which, though they may well make patients feel much better, do nothing to combat the cancer itself.

Most cancer patients welcome specific treatment, first and foremost because they hope it will overcome their disease, but also for the accompanying benefits: a sense of something positive being done, receiving care from expert professionals, an opportunity to meet other patients in a similar plight.

Many patients also dread anticancer treatment, some types of which have a fearsome reputation, justified to a greater or lesser extent.

All anticancer treatments have unwanted physical side-effects, whether temporary (nausea and vomiting after radiotherapy or chemotherapy) or permanent (mutilation after radical surgery), and these are often associated with psychological suffering. Treatment causes disruption to patients' lifestyle. It is expensive in terms of drugs and equipment and professional time. How far these drawbacks are justified must depend to a large extent on the aim of treatment.

Aims of Treatment

Anticancer treatment may be *curative, adjuvant* or *palliative.*

Curative treatment is intended to eliminate the cancer completely. While success in this goal can never be guaranteed, an excellent chance of achieving a cure exists in certain cases. Examples are surgery for localised bowel cancer, radiotherapy for some lymphomas, and cytotoxic chemotherapy for some leukaemias including the main childhood forms. Most cancer patients are prepared to tolerate very severe unwanted effects as the price of curing their disease, but there are limits to how much patients can endure, and also to how much their doctors are prepared to inflict upon them. Some radical surgical operations, entailing gross mutilation of the face or amputation of the lower half of the body, are seldom performed nowadays for this reason. However, research shows that many patients are willing, to a much greater extent than their doctors would expect, to undertake highly unpleasant treatments if there is even a small chance of a good response; and most patients claim no regrets about having treatment even if it has been an arduous experience with little obvious benefit.

Adjuvant treatment with chemotherapy or radiotherapy is intended to destroy any residual cancer cells left behind after the bulk of tumour has been surgically removed. Such treatment is likely to be helpful in selected cases only. Adjuvant radiotherapy reduces the risk of local recurrence; adjuvant chemotherapy delays the development of distant metastases, and thereby improves survival. Chemotherapy and radiotherapy used in adjuvant fashion have a rather different psychological impact from these same treatments used with curative or palliative intent, because there is no tangible benefit to balance out the negative aspects, and treatment may serve as a continual reminder of the risk of disease relapse.

Palliative treatment can often achieve worthwhile results even when a cancer is too advanced to be cured. Aims may include the relief of symptoms which are already present, prevention of symptoms which are highly likely to develop in the future, and/or the prolongation of life. Examples include surgical fixation of a pathological bone fracture; radiotherapy to a painful bone deposit or ulcerating skin lesion; chemotherapy to induce temporary shrinkage of a large tumour bulk. Palliative treatments should not be worse than the symptoms they are intended to control. Doses of radiotherapy and chemotherapy should be kept at the lowest effective level, to minimise side-effects, and regimes kept simple to avoid repeated treatment sessions. It is good practice to record both the aims and the results of treatment in the casenotes.

Introducing the Treatment

The prospect of starting a new treatment usually brings a mixture of hope and anxiety. The great majority of patients appreciate receiving full information beforehand. As well as what benefits to hope for, knowing what side-effects to expect is helpful for most. The risk that this strategy will cause suggestible patients to develop side-effects they might not otherwise have had, and scare others off treatment altogether, is relatively small.

A personal explanation of why a particular treatment is being recommended for the patient in question is essential in every case. Many patients are, however, so anxious during an important hospital consultation that they never take in the details of what they are told. A followup interview with a nurse who can explain things again, and answer questions which have occurred to the patient afterwards, is therefore most helpful.

If the proposed treatment is of a standard kind, various practical aids can be used as a supplement to (but *not* a substitute for) this individual interview. *Leaflets* may be written in a 'question and answer' format and include some photos or diagrams. *Videos* are especially helpful for children but also welcomed by many adults. Good leaflets and videos are not easy to produce, and it is worth seeking professional advice to achieve the optimum quality.

Introduction to a *'veteran patient'* who has undergone similar treatment in the past can have powerful effects, though not always of a desirable kind. Ex-patients who volunteer to counsel others should preferably be monitored by professional staff.

Research

Accurate information about the efficacy and acceptability of different treatments can only be gained through research, preferably in the form of randomised prospective clinical trials. Some apparently obvious assumptions have not been confirmed by research studies. For example, radical cancer operations such as mastectomy or limb amputation do not necessarily cause greater emotional distress than conservative treatments for the same conditions.

Some people shy away from the idea of carrying out research on patients with cancer, especially advanced cancer, fearing that 'experiments on the dying' will be deemed unethical. Such scruples are seldom justified, provided the research project concerned has proper scientific value and the patients' informed consent has been obtained. On the contrary, carrying out well-designed research is a much more 'ethical' activity than the common practice of choosing clinical treatments on the basis of either long-established habit, or the latest promotion from a drug company!

Many patients are only too pleased to take part in research studies. The knowledge that they are helping future sufferers, even if they derive no direct benefit themselves, may inject some worthwhile meaning into an otherwise dismal situation. Research subjects usually receive first-rate medical care because they have such frequent and thorough clinical assessments.

Quality of Life during Cancer Treatment (Clark and Fallowfield 1990; Slevin 1992)

Anticancer treatments used to be evaluated mainly in terms of *length* of survival, taking little account of *quality* of survival. Now, partly in recognition of the fact that some chemotherapy regimes have such unpleasant side-effects, systematic measures of *quality of life* are being introduced, both within formal protocols for clinical trials and in everyday clinical practice.

Various 'domains' can be measured: psychological, social, sexual, occupational, physical, spiritual, satisfaction with care. Trying to measure all of these in each patient is clearly over-ambitious. Indeed, measuring just one aspect is necessarily a crude approximation. Assessment instruments have to be quick and simple if they are to be given to large numbers of patients.

Many different assessment instruments are available (see Appendix on Measurement Scales). Some measure just one domain, for example the Karnofsky Scale measures physical functioning, and the Hospital Anxiety and Depression (HAD) Scale measures mood. Others, such as the Rotterdam Symptom Checklist, the Nottingham Health Profile and the Psychological Adjustment to Illness Scale (PAIS), provide a more global assessment. Alternative methods involve letting patients themselves choose a personal list of items which are important to them.

By definition, the concept of 'quality of life' is about the patient's own perceptions, and for this reason it is better to measure it with self-rating rather than observer-rating scales. Doctors' ratings of the severity of patients' symptoms, physical and psychological, fail to agree with patients' own ratings in a considerable proportion of cases.

Choice of Treatments

In many clinical situations there is no cut-and-dried 'best' treatment. For many cases of early breast cancer, for example, there is a choice between mastectomy, or local excision with adjuvant radiotherapy, with the chances of disease-free survival being much the same.

Doctors used to take treatment decisions on patients' behalf. This strategy is no longer widely acceptable. Current practice involves giving patients all the information available, and letting them decide for themselves what treatment—if any—they want.

Most patients welcome this opportunity for choice. Some have strong decided views. Others, though glad to have been consulted, will in fact ask the doctor to decide.

A few patients find the responsibility of choice a heavy burden at this time of crisis in their lives. This can be the case even for young, well-educated patients who might be expected—and often expect themselves—to assume control, but in fact suffer agonies of indecision.

Marion, a senior nurse in her 40s, developed a breast lump which was shown to be malignant on biopsy. Reading the medical literature on the various combinations of surgery, radiotherapy and chemotherapy in current use left her overwhelmed. She could not decide what treatment to have, and spent many weeks seeking second opinions from specialists around the country, before deciding on a simple mastectomy.

Patients who Refuse Treatment

In the days when a paternalistic medical profession dictated what was best for the patient, refusal of treatment was rather rare and when it did take place, sometimes led to a most unseemly show-down. As a junior doctor on a ward round, I remember one man asking the consultant if his operation might be postponed till after a booked holiday with his wife; the consultant turned red in the face and ordered the man to leave the hospital and not bother to come back. Nowadays, hopefully, such an incident would not occur.

There are many situations in which patient and/or doctor will quite reasonably decide that the side-effects and inconvenience of the proposed treatment are likely to outweigh its benefits, or more simply—in the case of advanced cancer when specific treatment can only delay the inevitable—that the time has come to stop. Even if patient and doctor do not quite agree on when this point has been reached, the doctor will usually respect the patient's wishes.

Occasionally, a patient refuses a treatment which in the doctor's opinion would have clearcut benefit. Although the patient's wishes must be given priority at the end of the day, it is always worth trying to explore the reasons behind a decision which appears misguided. They may prove perfectly rational and valid, but other possibilities would be:

- The patient is misinformed about the treatment. One man suffering from advanced carcinoma of the prostate had experienced horrible side-effects from radical pelvic irradiation in the past. He declined palliative radiotherapy to his painful bony metastases, until it was explained that the proposed low-dose treatment was unlikely to have any side-effects at all.

- The patient does not appreciate the likely consequences of *not* having treatment, for example a breast tumour may become ulcerated and infected if no local surgery or radiotherapy is given.
- Refusal of treatment, being likely to lead to an earlier death, is an easy way out of an unhappy life—a kind of passive suicide. Remediable factors may be present—a clinical depression responsive to psychotropic drugs, or miserable social circumstances which could be helped if they were disclosed.
- A statement of autonomy; refusal of treatment may be one of the few ways the patient can exert some control over an intolerable situation.

Conflicts can also arise when patients and their families—as opposed to patients and their doctors—hold different views about treatment. In theory, the views of the patient should carry most weight, though this principle may have to be modified if the patient is very old, very young or very ill. Sometimes the overbearing relative of a frail patient can browbeat doctors into either giving or withholding treatment against their better judgement.

Dependence on Treatment

As discussed above, many patients welcome specific treatment for their cancer, even if this causes marked side-effects without obvious benefit. The value of regular care and attention from expert professionals, hoping against hope for a last-minute response, or simply knowing that 'something is being done' or 'everything possible has been tried', is an important source of comfort for many patients and their families. Sometimes this means that the patient—or a relative—begs to persist with active treatment after the doctor considers there is no longer any value in doing so, and this can raise difficult issues about responsibility for decision-making and the use of resources.

Enid, aged 62, had metastatic breast cancer which was gradually advancing, and attended her local hospice as a day patient. She had taken tamoxifen for several years, but her consultant decided this drug was probably doing no good and might as well be stopped. Enid appeared to accept this, but then tearfully confided to one of the nurses that she did not feel safe without her tamoxifen. Over the next few weeks she continued to talk in the same vein, asking why other patients could have tamoxifen while she could not, and quoting articles she had read about the benefits of the drug. In view of the fact that tamoxifen is relatively free from side-effects, and also reasonably cheap, it was finally decided to reinstate the prescription and Enid became much happier although her disease continued to progress.

Withholding Specific Treatment

Withholding specific treatment altogether, for example in cases of inoperable lung cancer which is not causing much in the way of symptoms, can often be justified on the grounds that treatment would not prolong life, and might produce unpleasant side-effects. The danger is that lack of specific treatment can become equated with a general lack of communication and care.

Harry, aged 70, had been widowed just three weeks before he presented to his family doctor with cough and chest pain. Chest X-ray suggested lung cancer but bronchoscopy proved negative. No specific treatment was prescribed before his outpatient review three months later. Meanwhile, Harry was seen at home in the course of a research survey, and found to be deeply depressed. He attributed his depression primarily to missing his wife, and also to worsening pain in his ribs. He had not been back to his family doctor, nor asked for an earlier outpatient appointment. He said he guessed he had cancer, though 'The doctors have said nothing. They've got too many to see—they don't know or care about you as an individual. I don't mind if they tell me or not, it's up to them. I'm in the final chapter of my life, I believe—and hope.'

Patients who are not receiving specific treatment should be monitored frequently, so that new symptoms receive prompt attention and, equally important, they are not left feeling abandoned without psychological support.

SURGERY (Jacobsen and Holland 1989)

The trend in recent years has been away from radical cancer surgery, towards more limited excisions combined with adjuvant radiotherapy or chemotherapy. Even so, some tumours are still best treated by a major operation such as mastectomy, colostomy, hysterectomy with oophorectomy, laryngectomy, or amputation of a limb. Prophylactic surgery is occasionally recommended for patients with a strong family history of breast, colonic or ovarian cancer. Such procedures entail a permanent loss of body structure, body function, or both, and they understandably evoke much distress. However, the consequent mutilation or disablement usually seems the lesser of two evils if the alternative is unchecked progression of the cancer.

Worthwhile rehabilitation can often be achieved following a major operation for cancer. Breast reconstruction by plastic surgery gives excellent results for many mastectomy patients; failing this, the careful selection of prosthesis, bras and swimwear can make an important difference to activity and self-esteem. Other examples include restoration of speech after laryngectomy, and of mobility following an amputation. The skills of physiotherapists, occupational therapists, speech therapists, specialist nurses and other professionals have much to contribute here.

Before the Operation

Most patients feel anxious at the prospect of surgery. Even if the operation is to be a minor one, the process of admission to a hospital ward combined with various common fears—of not waking up after the anaesthetic, of something going wrong with the procedure, of postoperative pain—cause a certain amount of distress.

Most cancer operations cannot be described as 'minor', and the distress they cause is correspondingly greater. Uncertainty may contribute to this: wondering whether the tumour will prove to be more widespread than first thought, how large an operation will have to be done, or even whether the diagnosis actually is cancer at all. For example, till about ten years ago, women with breast lumps were managed by 'frozen section'; the patient remained under anaesthetic while the excised lump was examined by a pathologist and, if it proved malignant, a mastectomy was carried out right away. With modern techniques of investigation, accurate histology and staging are available before surgery, so that uncertainty of this kind can usually be avoided.

Occasionally, preoperative anxiety escalates out of control. Patients panic, cannot sleep, cause a disturbance on the ward, or refuse to go to the operating theatre at the last minute. A psychiatric consultation is often desirable in such cases. Thorough discussion may reveal the root of the patient's fears, for example they may reflect some former traumatic experience—heavy bleeding after previous surgery, somebody close having died on the operating table. Ventilation of past memories and present fears, combined with accurate information about the proposed operation, usually helps. Prescription of a benzodiazepine or neuroleptic drug is often indicated. Practical measures such as placing the patient first on the morning's list, allowing a relative to stay in the hospital the previous night, a move from open ward to single room or vice versa, may help the patient submit to surgery more calmly.

After the Operation

Relief, even euphoria, may supervene when the operation is safely over. Depressive reactions can, however, occur, especially if the patient has to be given bad news about the operative findings—for example if unsuspected liver metastases were found—or a valued body part has been removed.

Delirium (acute organic brain syndrome; confusional state) may develop postoperatively due to a metabolic disturbance or an adverse drug reaction, especially in older patients with pre-existing cognitive impairment, and in alcoholics.

Many patients are reluctant to look at their scar but it is usually advisable for them to do so earlier rather than later. This also applies to the spouse or partner.

Ways of Easing Adjustment to Surgery

• Preoperative counselling to make sure the patient understands the proposed procedure. Most cancer patients willingly accept a drastic operation if it offers the best chance of cure but a few are horrified at the prospect of, say, having a colostomy. Such patients may never be able to adjust psychologically if the surgery goes ahead. Their quality of life may be better with less radical treatment, even if the prognosis of their cancer is consequently less good.
• Preoperative training in anxiety management, for example using relaxation and imagery. Research studies have shown that such techniques can help reduce distress and pain before and after surgery.
• Postoperative counselling, often best carried out by an experienced nurse who is expert in the operation concerned and can follow up patients over a period of months, offering practical advice and an opportunity to ventilate emotions, and refer for specialised help more if problems develop.
• Peer support, perhaps from a self-help group. Witnessing first-hand the successful rehabilitation of a 'veteran' patient can have a tonic effect.

Surgeons

The personality of the surgeon can have a marked though sometimes unrecognised influence on patients' psychological adjustment. Those undergoing surgery tend to feel themselves in a passive, even child-like role, and to regard their surgeons as powerful authority figures. They develop strong emotions towards them, and invest their every word with great significance. This may be no bad thing if its general effect is to boost confidence in the surgeon; less good if the patient perceives the surgeon as a sadistic ogre! The phenomenon is a kind of 'transference' which may be especially strong when the surgeon has an obviously striking character, or when contact between patient and surgeon is too brief to permit a more realistic personal relationship to develop.

Similar things can of couse happen with doctors in other specialities, but the effect is especially marked with regard to surgeons.

CHEMOTHERAPY (Cull 1990; Holland and Lesko 1989)

Chemotherapy means drug treatment. In cancer work, the term is often used as shorthand for cytotoxic chemotherapy. Hormone therapy and immunotherapy can also be included under the 'chemotherapy' heading.

Cytotoxic Drugs

Cytotoxic drugs interfere with various stages of DNA synthesis or function. Leukaemias, lymphomas, testicular tumours, breast cancer and small cell (oat cell) lung cancer are among the most common of the many conditions for which they are used.

The several different types of drug act at different stages of cell division, and the most effective way to use them involves giving several types together: 'combination chemotherapy'. Treatment is usually divided into a number of doses (called 'pulses' or 'cycles') given every few weeks and often continuing for several months. Most cytotoxic drugs cannot be taken by mouth, only by intravenous injection.

Because cytotoxic drugs kill normal cells as well as cancer cells, they can have numerous side-effects including nausea and vomiting, diarrhoea, sore mouth, hair loss, tiredness, and bone marrow depression causing increased susceptibility to infections. Repeated injections are an ordeal for those patients who are afraid of needles or the sight of blood. The prolonged nature of the treatment, with pulses administered every three weeks or so for many months, means that patients are continually being reminded about their disease. Their lifestyle is disrupted because of the time and money spent on repeated visits to hospital, with consequent absences from home and work. Adjuvant chemotherapy, for example following surgery for early breast cancer, may be especially difficult to tolerate because there is no immediate benefit to make up for all these negative aspects. There is evidence from clinical trials that patients given adjuvant chemotherapy, especially if the course is a long one, suffer emotional distress over and above that normally associated with the diagnosis and treatment of cancer. Whether this is justified by their improved chances of longterm survival is probably an unanswerable question.

Chemotherapy given as primary treatment, and palliative chemotherapy to control the symptoms of advanced disease, both have a greater tangible benefit than adjuvant chemotherapy and the unwanted effects may therefore be more readily tolerated.

George, a married man of 40, became clinically depressed after receiving a diagnosis of small cell lung cancer. His main concern was that he would not live long enough to see his teenage son established in a career. He was glad to be offered palliative chemotherapy, and delighted to see the improvement on his chest X-ray. Though side-effects were quite severe, he accepted this: 'It's one week in three written off, but that's not too bad, considering what's wrong.' His depression resolved without specific treatment and he said he felt 'on top of the world' with renewed hope for the future.

Nausea and vomiting are among the most common and the most distressing of chemotherapy side-effects, although modern anti-emetic drugs have brought about greatly improved control. These symptoms are frequently exacerbated by *psychologically-based nausea and vomiting*, which affect up to 80% of patients receiving the more toxic chemotherapy regimes such as those containing cisplatin. The longer the course of treatment, the more common this problem becomes. Affected patients feel sick, or actually vomit, for several days prior to a planned treatment, in anticipation of what is to come. In others, the nausea or vomiting is triggered by a specific stimulus (cue) associated with chemotherapy; an example of Pavlovian conditioning. Sights, sounds or smells associated with treatment may act as cues, for example the disinfectant solution used to clean the skin before the injection, and the coffee served in the waiting room. Paradoxically, nausea and vomiting can even be triggered by things designed to prevent their occurrence, such as an anti-emetic tablet or a relaxation tape. Months or years after treatment has finished, some patients still feel sick when they encounter the stimulus concerned.

Clinical psychologists can help with such techniques as systemic desensitisation, guided imagery, progressive muscular relaxation and self-hypnosis. If nobody is available to teach such specialised techniques, commonsense measures include:

- Minimising waiting time before treatment.
- Minimising patients' bad expectations. Patients who are told to expect terrible nausea and vomiting, and patients who witness others being sick, are more likely to suffer badly when their time comes.
- Supportive counselling and a chance to ventilate anxieties.
- Distraction from cues: sucking mints to mask hospital smells and tastes, listening to music or relaxation tapes before treatment, performing mental tasks.

Hair loss matters greatly to some patients, whereas others do not mind too much wearing a wig, or even going bare-headed and making light of it.

> *Donna*, aged 38, was bald following her chemotherapy for lung cancer, except for a fluffy little 'top-knot' . For a while she wore a turban, but when the summer weather came she left this off, and made jokes about being 'a middle-aged punk'. She predicted that, on Christmas Day, she would tie a ribbon round her top-knot; this she did. A few days later she died.

Depression in chemotherapy patients may represent a reaction to the unpleasantness of the treatment, and/or result from the direct effects of cytotoxic drugs upon mood.

Rowena, a happily married 45-year-old woman whose life re-volved around her home and the care of her family, was receiving adjuvant chemotherapy with CMF (cyclophosphamide, metho-trexate and 5-FU) following the local excision of a malignant breast lump. A day or two after each pulse of treatment she became low in mood, tearful, panicky and tremulous with a heavy feeling in the chest. Even at other times she felt depressed, especially in the mornings, though her sleep and appetite were not impaired. At interview, her main concern was the fear that recurrence and death might separate her from her dearly-loved family. After several weeks' treatment with amitriptyline 100 mg at night, and three sessions of supportive discussion with a psychiatrist, Rowena's mood had improved greatly. It was impossible to tell how far this improvement resulted from the psychiatric interven-tion, as opposed to the coincidental ending of the course of chemotherapy. The timing of symptoms in her case is strongly suggestive of some direct effect of chemotherapy upon mood, but the psychological impact of the cancer diagnosis was also import-ant.

Organic brain syndromes causing confusion or disturbed behaviour have been reported during cytotoxic drug treatment, with vincristine, vinblastine and L-asparaginase being especially implicated, but are not a major problem in clinical practice.

Longterm effects of chemotherapy include infertility, pulmonary fibrosis, cardiomyopathy, cognitive impairments and the induction of second malignancies. Most longterm survivors of cytotoxic treatment are superficially well-adjusted but some are prone to chronic anxiety about possible relapse of their cancer.

Hormone (Endocrine) Therapy

Steroids such as prednisolone and dexamethasone are widely used in cancer treatment. Often combined with other drugs, they are specifically indicated for lymphomas and leukaemias and for myeloma. Steroids are also useful for symptom control in many kinds of cancer: for the reduction of oedema, for example in cerebral tumours and spinal cord compression; to reduce nausea and vomiting in patients on cytotoxic drugs; and, in advanced cancer, to promote wellbeing and uplifting of mood. In 5-10% of cases, steroids induce more drastic mental changes than the mild euphoria which is intended. Mood changes (mania or depression or a mixture of the two), paranoid psychosis or delirium are recognised complications of steroid therapy, and usually occur within a few days of starting the drug or increasing the dose. Patients with a past psychiatric history may be most at risk. In the event of an extreme psychiatric reaction, it is usually necessary to discontinue the steroid, or at least reduce the dose, and consider adding a psychotropic drug, either a neuroleptic or an antidepressant depending on the symptoms.

Steroids taken for any length of time produce characteristic bodily changes: a moon-shaped face, weight gain on the trunk but wasting of the limbs, acne or striae on the skin. Many patients are self-conscious about their altered appearance, and other people, taking steroid-induced weight gain for a sign of good health, may make unwittingly hurtful remarks.

Sex hormone manipulation is used for some tumours, most commonly cancers of the breast and prostate. Removal of ovaries or testicles, medication to block sex hormone function, or administration of hormones of the opposite sex, are among the procedures used. The psychological consequences of amenorrhoea, growth of body hair, and deepening of the voice in women, and of impotence and breast enlargement in men, are naturally distressing. Fortunately, the drugs now available for firstline treatment (such as tamoxifen for breast cancer, gonadotrophin-releasing blockers for prostatic cancer) are relatively free of such effects.

RADIOTHERAPY (Holland 1989b)

Radiotherapy is the use of high-energy irradiation to destroy unwanted tissue, and its main use is in the treatment of cancer. *Radical* radiotherapy, given with the aim of cure, is the treatment of choice for some cancers which are highly sensitive to radiation (for example the early stages of laryngeal cancer and of Hodgkin's disease), or those which would be difficult or impossible to remove surgically because of their position in the body (for example lung cancer growing close to the mediastinum). *Adjuvant* radiotherapy is used to reduce the risk of local recurrence after limited surgery, most commonly for cancer of the breast. *Palliative* radiotherapy, which forms a large part of the work of any radiotherapy department, often brings worthwhile benefits like controlling pain from bone metastases, and is sometimes indicated on an emergency basis for shrinking a tumour mass in cases of superior vena cava obstruction (SVCO) or incipient paraplegia.

The Radiotherapy Process

Most radiotherapy is delivered by an external beam. Radical or adjuvant treatments are divided into a number of fractions spread over several weeks, because giving the total dose at once would cause too much damage to healthy tissue. For palliative radiotherapy, the total dose is smaller and can sometimes be given in two or three fractions or even just one.

The actual treatment process causes no pain, indeed there is nothing to feel at all, but some patients are frightened by the prospect of having to lie quite still, alone in the treatment room, underneath a formidable-looking machine. Most of them soon get used to this, especially if they have had a proper introductory explanation of radiotherapy and have been allowed to look at the equipment, or see a video, before their own treatment begins. Patients with claustrophobic tendencies, however, may find radiotherapy a great ordeal. Ways of helping such patients to tolerate radiotherapy include administration of a short-acting tranquilliser before each treatment session, and psychological techniques similar to those described above for management of anticipatory nausea and vomiting in patients on chemotherapy.

Less often, radiotherapy is delivered by implants of radioactive material left inside the tumour for a few hours or days. Patients must be nursed in relative isolation while such implants are in place.

Many people have a dread of radiotherapy, because they associate the word with incurable cancer, and also because they are frightened of radioactivity and may harbour unfounded fears about its effects. One patient would not let her grandchildren come near her because she believed, wrongly, that a course of external beam radiotherapy to her abdomen some years before had rendered her permanently radioactive and a danger to their health.

Side-effects of Radiotherapy

Side-effects of radiotherapy arise because healthy cells are destroyed as well as cancer cells. The nature and severity of side-effects depend on the dose given, and the part of the body treated. High-dose radiotherapy to any area may cause soreness of the skin, tiredness and general malaise. Treatment to the upper abdomen often causes nausea; treatment to the lower abdomen or pelvis often causes diarrhoea; treatment to the head often causes hair loss. Whereas radical courses inevitably cause some side-effects, however, palliative regimes may have none at all. Any side-effects tend to build up during the course of treatment, usually reaching their maximum severity a week or so after the course is finished, before gradually clearing up. This delayed toxicity should be carefully explained to patients, otherwise they will assume the treatment has been a failure or even made them worse.

Patients who survive months or years after high-dose radiotherapy may develop longterm side-effects, often due to fibrosis of the treated area. Permanent cognitive impairment may follow irradiation of the brain; permanent sterility may follow treatment of the gonads.

Whether radiotherapy can directly cause depression is not clearly established, though some patients do describe lowered mood in association with this treatment.

Rex, in his late 40s, had felt depressed for a year before his inoperable lung cancer was diagnosed. He put the depression down to the 'anguish' of being unemployed for the first time in his life. He was given a course of radiotherapy to relieve the pain in his chest. He said of the treatment: 'I found it very, very hard to cope with, but I got through because they'd warned me what to expect. All the energy drained out of me afterwards, and then the tears broke.' By the end of the course, however, his pain had improved 'like a miracle' and his depressive symptoms had lifted.

COMPLEMENTARY THERAPIES (Holland, Geary and Furman 1989)

Acupuncture, aromatherapy, healing, herbalism, homeopathy, hypnotherapy, reflexology and visualisation are examples of complementary therapies. 'Complementary' is a better term than 'alternative' because most practitioners recommend these treatments be used as well as orthodox (conventional) medical ones, not instead of them.

Complementary therapies are occasionally used in National Health Service (NHS) settings, but for the most part they are delivered in the private sector by practitioners without a medical qualification. The use of complementary therapies by cancer patients in Western society is probably increasing, the best-known venue in Britain being the Bristol Cancer Help Centre. The recommended package usually includes some combination of both practical and psychological techniques.

The use of complementary therapies in cancer patient care may excite controversy. Some people are passionately convinced of their value, while others dismiss them as useless and even dangerous mumbo-jumbo. As yet, there is no sound proof that complementary therapies improve either length of survival or quality of life for patients with cancer. It is, however, fair to say that no proper clinical trials on this subject have been done.

Attractions of Complementary Therapies

Why are complementary therapies increasingly popular? Some of the practical aspects, for example massage with fragrant oils, are pleasant in themselves. When delivered by a sympathetic therapist, they naturally help to make patients feel valued and cared for.

To some extent this reflects badly on orthodox medicine. Many medical and surgical treatments for cancer, besides producing unpleasant physical side-effects, are delivered in a busy 'high-tech' hospital environment where patients are sometimes justified in feeling that staff have neither the time nor the interest to relate to them on a personal level.

Orthodox treatments also have the more subtle disadvantage of placing patients in a passive role. Apart from attending hospital and obeying instructions, patients themselves have little scope for taking part in a way that will maximise their chances of a good response. Complementary therapies, in contrast, encourage patient participation. Despite the lack of proof that a vegetarian diet, a daily meditation session or a change in mental attitude really will improve prognosis of their cancer, many patients find such lifestyle changes give them positive goals to strive for, and instill a fresh sense of hope.

Drawbacks of Complementary Therapies

Complementary therapies, like any others, may cause ill-effects if practised inappropriately; or when patients themselves invest too much faith in them.

Most complementary therapists have good intentions and a genuine belief in the value of their methods, misguided though such belief may sometimes be. A minority are unscrupulous charlatans who deliberately exploit vulnerable cancer patients for their own gratification or for financial gain.

It is sad when patients, desperately trying to deny that their cancer is incurable, spend most of their remaining time, money and energy on complementary therapy which is doomed to fail; and then, when forced to accept that their cancer is progressing after all, perhaps blame themselves for not trying hard enough.

Even sadder are those few patients whose cancers might well have been cured by orthodox medicine but reject this in favour of a complementary approach which does not cure.

Some kinds of complementary therapy, though 'natural', can be harmful especially if used to excess. Examples are strict diets which, besides being arduous to follow, lead to nutritional deficiencies; and certain herbal remedies which are toxic to the liver.

Finding a Balance

Fortunately, it seems that both orthodox and complementary practitioners are now becoming more willing to work together and learn from each other. Some NHS centres are introducing complementary techniques alongside conventional ones; and some complementary therapists have agreed to submit their methods to controlled clinical trials.

Complementary therapy cannot provide the miracle cures which some enthusiasts claim, but may well have more modest benefits to offer. Individual complementary methods remain to be evaluated. Meanwhile, the overall philosophy of a 'whole-person' approach, in which patients themselves are invited to play an active part, has a widespread and valid appeal.

FURTHER READING

Clark AW, Fallowfield, LJ (1990) Quality of life measurements in patients with malignant disease: a review. *Journal of the Royal Society of Medicine 79* 165–9

Cull A (1990) Invited review: psychological aspects of cancer and chemotherapy. *Journal of Psychosomatic Research 34* 129–40

Holland JC. Fears and abnormal reactions to cancer in physically healthy individuals. In Holland JC, Rowland JH (eds) (1989a) *Handbook of Psychooncology.* Oxford University Press: New York

Holland JC. Radiotherapy. In Holland JC, Rowland JH (eds) (1989b) *Handbook of Psychooncology.* Oxford University Press: New York

Holland JC, Lesko LM. Chemotherapy, endocrine therapy and immunotherapy. In Holland JC, Rowland JH (eds) (1989) *Handbook of Psychooncology.* Oxford University Press: New York

Holland JC, Geary N, Furman A. Alternative cancer therapies. In Holland JC, Rowland JH (eds) (1989) *Handbook of Psychooncology.* Oxford University Press: New York

Jacobsen P, Holland JC. Psychological reactions to cancer surgery. In Holland JC, Rowland JH (eds) (1989) *Handbook of Psychooncology.* Oxford University Press: New York

Slevin ML (1992) Quality of life: philosophical question or clinical reality? *British Medical Journal 305* 466–9

Wardle J, Pope R (1992) The psychological costs of screening for cancer. *Journal of Psychosomatic Research 36* 609–24

2
Models of Psychological Response

This part of the book begins with an overview of the various losses which cancer can inflict on patients' and their families' lives. Some of the theoretical models which seek to explain how patients cope with life-threatening illness will then be outlined.

The intention is to describe a range of psychological responses, without dividing them into 'normal' and 'abnormal', or 'good' and 'bad'. Though some types of response do tend to get labelled as superior to others, value-judgements are seldom constructive. Always ask 'Does this response suit this patient?' rather than 'How would *I* react in this situation?' or 'What *should* a patient in this situation do and feel?' Some responses, of course, are clearly not desirable because they lead to increased suffering for the patient or of others; these will be considered in the next section.

CANCER AND LOSS

Cancer may affect the emotions in many complex ways, and no single model could embrace them all. However, many of cancer's psychological effects can be understood in terms of reaction to *loss*—or the threat of loss in the future.

Loss of physical strength and wellbeing is most keenly felt, even in the early stages of illness, by patients with manual jobs and those who enjoy sport or practical hobbies.

When and if physical weakness becomes so marked as to cause *loss of independence*, almost all patients feel frustrated by their enforced inactivity. Many feel concerned or guilty about being a burden to relatives or staff, however willing to look after them these carers may be. Of all the practical deprivations, giving up driving the car is the one which comes hardest of all to many patients in the modern Western world.

Loss of role can lead to boredom, and perhaps cause friction with other people who have had to take over the patient's former duties. In one survey, a high proportion of patients with advanced cancer said that 'not being able to do things' was the worst aspect of their illness.

Loss of interpersonal relationships is by no means universal, because many relationships become deepened and enhanced through the experience of cancer. However, problems in relationships do commonly occur. When it comes to talking about the distressing topic of serious and possibly fatal illness, *communication barriers* may develop even within the closest families. Some patients also suffer communication problems due to the physical effects of their condition, for example laryngectomy patients whose speech cannot be understood, or brain tumour patients who cannot find the words they want.

Some cancer patients describe a sense of *alienation* from people in good health: one woman said of her family 'All the rest of them are normal and I'm the freak.'

Loss of sexual function can be distressing at any age, and *loss of fertility* for younger patients.

Loss of physical integrity includes obvious changes in outward appearance and impairment of bodily functions, also the more subtle losses covered by the phrase 'body image'. Body weight is often altered; a wasted body proclaims the diagnosis of serious illness in cruelly obvious fashion, whereas in other cases weight gain (often due to medication with steroids) gives a misleading illusion of wellbeing. A few patients have obvious visible deformities due to their cancer or its treatment, for example lesions on the face. Many other common changes such as colostomy, mastectomy, or baldness due to chemotherapy can easily be concealed from the casual observer, yet some patients are excruciatingly self-conscious about them. Others do not mind so much, like the breast cancer patient who wrote after her mastectomy: 'There's more to life than a beautiful body—cancer taught me that.'

Loss of life expectancy can induce profound sadness or anger, even for some patients who are already quite elderly. Existing goals for the future may have to be modified, or replaced by more modest ones. Many patients can talk openly about such matters, and acknowledge the threat through practical actions such as making a will. For others, the prospect of death and dying—encroaching loss of independence and dignity, separation from their loved ones, wondering what the mode of their death will be and if any afterlife awaits them—are too threatening to contemplate. Such patients' suppressed fears are sometimes manifest through dreams.

Loss of control—lack of opportunity for personal influence over the disease process—is important for some. Newly diagnosed patients may feel shaken, almost affronted, to realise that their bodies had been harbouring a growing cancer without their knowledge for months or years. A quest for meaning in the illness may or may not yield an explanation which brings comfort or makes sense. The fear that cancer could strike again, apparently at random, at any time and in any organ, may be a potent source of anxiety even for those who appear to have been cured. With certain illnesses, for example diabetes or cardiovascular disease, changes in lifestyle can be shown to influence prognosis. This is less true for cancer. Many patients feel like passive victims, as much at the mercy of powerful medical treatments as of the disease itself.

Loss of mental integrity—unfamiliar emotions, behaviour which is out of character, failing intellectual powers—seem to threaten the very essence of personality. Such changes usually occur early on for patients with primary brain tumours, are a common feature of secondary brain tumours (cerebral metastases), and may also result from disturbances in body chemistry or the side-effects of certain drugs. When patients themselves are not aware of these changes, they may be all the more disturbing for the relatives.

All the losses may seem overwhelming, especially for younger patients, yet most do manage to cope.

Andrew, aged 27, had had his right leg amputated because of osteosarcoma of the femur. He seemed to adapt quite calmly to the dual psychological traumas of diagnosis of life-threatening illness and the loss of a limb. He resumed his career in journalism, and got married. Five years later he developed metastases in his lungs. He accepted chemotherapy, but was well aware this treatment would not cure his disease. He made a new will and put his affairs carefully in order.

Accompanying the over-riding threat of inevitable loss of life, Andrew had lost much else. He had to give up his job, and his car, both of which had meant much to him. At home, confined to bed all day, he tried to keep up with current affairs through radio and TV, but found it difficult to concentrate. His devoted wife looked after him well, but Andrew knew that her own career prospects were suffering on his account, and felt bad about this. He regretted the end of their sexual relationship, and the knowledge they would never have any children. He said he felt 'like a tree cut down in its prime.'

Andrew went through a phase of upsetting his wife by remarks like 'Why not ditch me and go for a job in London—you'll soon find yourself another bloke up there.' Brief counselling enabled both partners to understand that such outbursts were an expression of Andrew's frustration and anger at his own condition, and resentment of his wife's success and good health. In discussion, Andrew revealed fears that his concentration difficulties resulted from cerebral metastases. Normal neurological examination and normal CT scan of his brain dispelled this fear and, once he stopped worrying about it so much, his concentration improved. He acknowledged that current affairs were perhaps no longer of much relevance to him. Andrew spent the remaining weeks of his life in reasonable spirits, listening to music programmes, his dog lying for long hours at the foot of his bed.

FACTORS WHICH INFLUENCE RESPONSE (Holland 1989; Rowland 1989a)

No two patients with cancer show exactly the same emotional response, even if their physical status is very similar. Response depends on the individual perception of the threat of cancer, which is determined by the characteristics of the person concerned.

The Personal Meaning of Illness

'What does this illness mean to this person?' is often a useful starting-point for understanding a patient's response. Nobody can predict the answer to this question with any confidence for any individual—including themselves. However, certain features of that individual may help to suggest what the answer will be.

The most obvious interpretations of a cancer diagnosis are negative ones—a loss, a threat, a punishment. Their unfavourable impact is likely to be especially marked for patients with other risk factors such as social isolation, low socioeconomic status, past history of psychiatric illness, alcohol or drug abuse, other recent life stresses, and a tendency to be rigid and pessimistic in outlook. Striking exceptions are sometimes seen, however, when a diagnosis of cancer seems to enable a patient to transcend longstanding emotional maladjustment.

Ronald, a clerk aged 60, was recently divorced and had many years' history of heavy drinking and recurrent depression, having once tried to kill himself using car exhaust fumes. He presented to the chest clinic with one year's history of tiredness and cough. Squamous cell lung cancer was diagnosed, and treated by surgery. Two months later his depression was much improved, he had given up drinking and smoking and become reunited with his wife.

Many patients see positive aspects to their illness as well as the negative ones; for example it may represent a challenge to be fought and overcome.

Others are not unduly distressed by learning they have cancer. In the case of, say, an elderly widow(er) whose main goals in life have been accomplished, this response merits respect; for a younger person to welcome cancer as a natural way out of an unhappy life situation or state of mind is equally understandable but perhaps should not be taken at face value.

A few patients positively welcome the 'sick role' as bringing practical benefits like early retirement or rehousing, care and attention from family and friends, and release from unwelcome obligations.

Age

Beliefs about how people of different ages react to cancer are not always backed up by factual data. There is some evidence that younger patients suffer more emotional distress, which makes intuitive sense because young ones have more to lose. Besides the prospect of their life expectancy being greatly curtailed, they face being denied many of the experiences which most people take for granted: pursuing a career, getting married, having children and seeing them grow up. Older patients, already nearing the end of their natural lifespan and having already had the chance to achieve their goals, might be expected to react with greater equanimity. However, older patients do face some special problems. Cancer holds great stigma and fear for some of them, and this may lead to long delay in presentation of symptoms, or denial of the diagnosis. They may already be lonely, impoverished and unhappy in reaction to the usual losses of old age: death of relatives and friends, retirement, physical frailty.

It is unwise to make generalised assumptions based on age. Many elderly women, for example, are greatly distressed by 'body image' change after mastectomy, even though their lifestyle no longer includes sexual activity or wearing low-cut clothes. Old age in itself need not be a bar to the successful treatment of cancer; my own mother-in-law, aged 93, has made an excellent recovery from bowel cancer surgery last year.

Sex

Psychiatric symptoms of depression and anxiety are more common in female cancer patients than male ones. Suicide, however, occurs more often in males. These sex differences parallel those found in the general population. Maybe men are less likely to admit to emotional problems; research shows that female cancer patients tend to describe their main concerns in psychological terms, whereas men more often cite practical matters. There is also some evidence that men make greater use of denial, while women take a more realistic view. Individual variation is so wide, however, that generalisations based on the patient's sex are not particularly helpful in clinical practice.

Religious Belief

An active religious belief tends to go along with good adaptation to illness but the effect is not perhaps such a strong one as might be expected. Many religious people derive comfort from their faith, or believe their suffering serves a purpose. A few lose their faith after becoming ill, feeling that God has abandoned them. In contrast, having cancer may lead some non-believers to God, or prompt a conversion from one faith to another.

Past Experience of Cancer

A patient who has seen relatives or friends die from cancer is likely to respond rather differently from one who has witnessed successful responses to treatment in other people. Some patients, though having no direct experience of cancer in their own personal circle, have been deeply influenced by portrayals of the illness in novels, plays or documentaries. Many lay people, unaware that the term 'cancer' covers a multitude of conditions with differing effects, use such experiences as the basis of generalised assumptions which do not apply to their own case.

Past Psychiatric History

Patients who have suffered from depression, anxiety or other psychiatric problems at any time in the past are at risk of relapsing under the stress of having cancer. Looking at this question the other way round, a high proportion of those cancer patients who become severely depressed give a past history of depression. Again, individual case histories prove exceptions.

Jo, a 66-year-old married storeman, had suffered from continuous depression and anxiety for many years. He developed a cough and lost weight, and was found to have small cell lung cancer. He said he was told 'It can't be cured but we can shrivel it up for twelve months or so.'

After two cycles of cytotoxic chemotherapy, his physical symptoms had improved and his depression had gone. He said 'I couldn't have had better treatment if I'd been a millionaire. If I've only got twelve months they're going to be happy ones.'

Cultural Attitudes

Attitudes to cancer vary around the world, also between different sections of society within the same country.

In Britain, until about twenty years ago—and in many other countries even today—the diagnosis was usually concealed from the patient because cancer carried so much stigma, and implied such a grim prognosis. Relatives might be told while the patient was kept in ignorance. The situation in Britain has changed so much that it will be assumed in this book that the patient has been told the truth.

Current Life Circumstances

The effect of these often 'cuts both ways'. Happily married patients, for example, benefit from their spouse's help in withstanding the stress of their illness, yet also have more to lose if they should not survive. In general, however, good *social support* can provide a 'buffer' against the adverse psychological impact of stressful events such as developing cancer.

Personality

The concept of 'personality', which refers to relatively enduring psychological characteristics of the individual, is an important one but difficult to define or measure. Personality variables are not rigidly fixed; sometimes the same individual reacts in contrasting ways in different situations or at different times of life. The ability to be flexible in outlook and behaviour appears to be helpful in coping with the stress of becoming a cancer patient. So does the ability to take an active, confrontational stance towards the illness. People possessing traits of the so-called 'hardy personality'—the trio of 'challenge, commitment and control'—are well-equipped. A related concept is 'locus of control'. Patients with an 'internal' locus, who are ready to take personal responsibility for their own state of health, tend to make a happier emotional adjustment than those with an 'external' locus, who tend to rely on the professionals or on Fate.

The following few pages will give an outline of some theoretical models of adjustment to cancer, first using some terms and concepts from modern health psychology, and then from a more traditional psychodynamic perspective. These are just two of the systems which those of different professional backgrounds have found useful in explaining and classifying their patients' reactions.

ATTITUDES AND COPING STYLES

Classifying Mental Attitude to Cancer

Steven Greer and his colleagues in London, working primarily with breast cancer patients, have described the following categories:

- *Fatalism* (previously called *stoic acceptance*) is the most common. Patients acknowledge the seriousness of their illness but accept it as their lot, with little or no show of emotional distress, and carrying on their lives much as before.

  'I know it's cancer but I can't do much about it, so there's no point getting upset.'

- *Positive avoidance* (previously called *denial*) involves 'playing down' the threat of the illness.

'They haven't said what's wrong but it's probably nothing much anyway.'

Often this seems to be a quite successful way of coping, though more extreme degrees of denial can cause problems.
* *Helplessness–hopelessness* refers to a passive 'giving-up' in the face of the cancer. Patients feel overwhelmed by their illness and make little effort to cope or adjust. They usually go along with whatever treatment is recommended but take no initiative of their own, for example not reporting a new symptom unless specifically asked about it. They may abandon their work and their hobbies long before advancing disease forces them to do so.

'I can't see any future, this seems like the end of the world.'

It is important to rule out a treatable depressive illness in patients who present a helpless--hopeless attitude.
* *Fighting spirit* patients rise to the challenge of overcoming cancer. They find out as much as possible about their condition, demand a say in choice of treatment, and often seek out complementary therapies in which they themselves can take an active role, for example adopting a new diet or exercise regime or undertaking a course of psychotherapy. They are resolved to live as fully as possible, often aiming towards defined practical goals.   One patient said 'I'm determined to live for my daughter's wedding.' His daughter was three years old.
* *Anxious preoccupation* is self-explanatory. Patients, even if objectively in remission, are constantly thinking about cancer, and interpret every minor physical change as a sign of relapse.

Some research studies have found that patients with a 'fighting spirit' tend to live longer than others, whereas the prognosis for 'helpless–hopeless' patients is particularly poor. It is, however, always difficult to be sure of the direction of cause and effect in studies of this kind; some 'helpless–hopeless' patients may already have occult advanced disease which is why they feel so weak and low in the first place, whereas those in good general condition can better summon up a 'fighting spirit' response.

Encouraging a fighting spirit is currently fashionable, but this strategy does not suit every patient's personality, and some will be made miserable and ill-at-ease if it is forced upon them, and guilty if the disease continues to advance ('I'm afraid my attitude wasn't positive enough.')

While placing any given patient into one of these categories is a neat, easily-understood method, it is probably an oversimplification, as many show a mixture of attitudes which may alter over time. A better approach is to construct an individual profile depending on how much of each attitude the patient shows. A questionnaire, the MAC (Mental Attitude to Cancer) Scale, exists for this purpose.

Coping Styles (Rowland 1989b)

Much psychological research in recent years has examined the 'coping styles' of people under stress. Using brief definitions:

- 'Stress' results when the demands on a person exceed his or her capacity to respond.
- 'Coping' refers to strategies for dealing with stress. These include cognitions (for example, putting the illness to the back of one's mind) and/or practical behaviours (for example, talking to friends).

Patients who are coping successfully are not overwhelmed by emotional distress—though such distress is not abolished completely. They can change their lifestyle to adapt to physical handicaps. They can maintain their own sense of self-worth, and their relationships with others.

Common successful coping strategies include:

- *Avoidance*: many patients, though well aware of the nature of their illness, resolve not to dwell on the subject. They concentrate on keeping busy and carrying on as normal, and manage to push cancer to the back of their minds. Reminders of illness—hospital visits, TV programmes or magazine features, casual remarks by other people—may upset them.
- *Mastery*: some patients achieve a sense of mastery by being able to attribute their illness to a specific cause, and identify active steps they can take to keep healthy in future. Their outlook is

through rose-coloured spectacles; while aware that some patients with a similar condition will relapse and die, they assume that they themselves will fall into the good-prognosis category, justifying this by statements like 'I was lucky, mine was caught early.'

- *Positive appraisal*: many patients previously treated for cancer, once having had time to overcome their initial distress, report some psychological benefits. In one of my own research series, 155 breast cancer patients who remained well two years after diagnosis were asked to describe the ways in which their outlook on life had been altered by their illness experience. Two-thirds reported some sustained change in attitude, this change being rated in positive terms by all but a few. Many patients spoke of an increased appreciation of life, and a better capacity for living in the present; less concern about trivial matters, and setting less store by material possessions; greater self-confidence, and greater willingness to fufil their own wishes rather than give in to other people. Typical quotations included:

'I've got my priorities straight now.'

'Getting new carpets or a new car isn't really important.'

'Now I do what *I* want to do.'

'Every day is a bonus.'

'Things are so beautiful—I don't take this world for granted any more.'

PSYCHODYNAMIC MODELS: MENTAL DEFENCE MECHANISMS

'Psychodynamic' models have evolved from the psychoanalytic theories of Sigmund Freud (1856–1939). They offer one line of approach to understanding emotions and behaviour, both normal and pathological, and form the basis of many present-day schools of psychotherapy.

Psychodynamic theory is too complicated to explain in any detail here, but a central principle is that experiences and relationships of early childhood, combined with instinctive drives, continue to influence a person's feelings and behaviour throughout adult life. This influence is largely unconscious, but may be explored by examining such things as the quirks of everyday conduct, the content of dreams, and the 'transference' towards a psychotherapist.

Parts of psychodynamic theory are helpful in understanding emotional response to cancer, as outlined below. Psychodynamic *therapy* for cancer patients will be considered later in the book.

Some enthusiasts seek to explain the onset of cancer itself in psychodynamic terms. Explanations of this kind can never be proved or disproved. Some are frankly bizarre; for example, one psychoanalyst explained a tumour on a young man's neck as a 'symbolic representation of his repressed wish to become pregnant'! Such interpretations seem more likely to be distressing than helpful to patients. On occasion, it is true, a skilled therapist is able to propose a psychodynamic model which, by placing the illness in the context of the individual's life history, adds some worthwhile sense of meaning to the cancer experience. In general, however, this approach is out of fashion and probably rightly so.

Psychodynamic models of *reaction* to cancer are also slightly oldfashioned, but can still be useful. One relevant Freudian concept is the set of *mental (or ego) defence mechanisms*. These are theoretical unconscious processes designed to protect against anxiety. Their operation can often be clearly seen in daily life, and they provide an explanantion for many common reaction patterns in cancer patients, their relatives and staff. A selection of defence mechanisms is listed below.

- *Denial*: the best-known one, which often serves a useful purpose but can cause problems if taken to extremes. Denial will be discussed in more detail later.
- *Projection*: attributing one's own unacknowledged emotions to other people. Patients often become irritable with their relatives because they are not aware of their own sadness, fear or anger regarding their disease.
- *Displacement*: redirecting emotions from their real object towards another which is easier to cope with. The father of a

young man who was dying from a lymphoma seldom came to visit his son, but had recently become a volunteer fund-raiser for a cancer charity and spent long hours on this work.

- *Sublimation*: channelling unacceptable primitive emotions into a more edifying outlet. The classic example would be diversion of frustrated sexual energy into artistic creation, good works or religious zeal.
- *Regression*: a return to an earlier stage of psychological maturity. This can be seen in patients of all ages who become child-like and dependent when they are ill.
- *Intellectualisation*: emphasising reason and factual knowledge, at the expense of emotional aspects. One highly intelligent young couple devoted themselves to an extensive study of the relevant medical literature when the husband developed a rare form of cancer. However, they never spoke of their feelings about his disease, nor of the possibility that he would not get better.
- *Conversion*: the expression of unacknowledged emotional distress in the guise of a physical symptom. This can be especially difficult to recognise when it occurs in a patient already known to have a serious illness.

The following story illustrates the application of mental mechanisms and simple psychodynamic concepts to one cancer patient's case.

Albert, a 65-year-old retired gardener who lived with his wife Della and three of their six grown-up children, presented with an acute chest infection and was admitted to hospital. Investigations revealed inoperable lung cancer (squamous cell). While Albert remained very ill, the ward doctor apparently told Della his diagnosis, and said he would probably live only two or three weeks. This medical prediction proved wrong; Albert improved and went home. Because Della was unsure what Albert himself had been told of the diagnosis, and because he never talked about the matter, she did not raise the topic with him.

continued

continued

(This part of the story illustrates the communication barriers between husband and wife which are quite common when one partner has cancer. Also, it shows that for a doctor or nurse to pronounce on life expectancy often proves a mistake. Albert's silence could be construed as evidence of denial and this is indeed one explanation. Alternatively, he may have made a conscious decision not to discuss his illness—suppression—or he may be genuinely ignorant of what is wrong.)

Six months later Albert was referred to the Day Centre at his local hospice, because his family were finding it hard to cope. His physical condition appeared reasonably good, with little deterioration shown on his chest X-ray. However, at each attendance he asked to see the doctor because of a fresh complaint; nausea one day, back pain the next, then headache. Repeated physical examinations and investigations revealed no obvious cause for these symptoms. Several staff said they found Albert a difficult patient. He came over as an inarticulate man whose conversation was limited to practical matters such as what time his transport would come and what was for pudding that day. He would spend his time at the Day Centre lying on the bed, claiming he was not well enough take part in any of the structured activities, though at weekends he was known to travel considerable distances to caravan rallies, driven by one of his sons.

(Although Albert has a genuine life-threatening illness, it does seem likely that his multiple bodily complaints are at least in part of psychological origin. He is expressing his unacknowledged emotional distress through somatisation—using the mental mechanism of conversion. He is provoking various negative feelings in the doctors and nurses. They may be frustrated at their inability to find physical explanations and treatments for his various presenting complaints—displeased that Albert rejects the Day Centre facilities in favour of his own weekend hobbies—and guilty because they and their colleagues have not managed to adequately address the question of diagnosis and prognosis with Albert. In finding him 'difficult', they may be projecting onto him their own feelings of inadequacy.)

At this stage Albert was referred for a psychiatric assessment. No evidence of clinical depression, or other formal psychiatric illness, was found. Asked what he had been told about his physical diagnosis, Albert skirted round the topic in vague terms, saying 'It's like a hernia on the chest—the future's uncertain.'

continued

continued

Asked about his personal history, Albert described a most unhappy childhood in which both he and his mother had been dominated, and frequently beaten, by the alcoholic man he assumed to be his father. At the age of eleven he discovered his birth certificate, which indicated he was actually another man's son—a discovery which had greatly perplexed him ever since. He could not bring himself to ask his mother about the matter until ten years later, when she was dying of cancer. His raising of the topic at that point, far from resolving the issue, provoked a distressing deathbed scene. Albert never did establish his father's identity. During the interview he stated several times 'I wish I could know my true name.' Albert left home early to get married, but repeated the pattern of drinking and violence towards his own wife and children for a number of years before 'mellowing' in middle life. He admitted he had been 'the very devil' to his family, but stressed that he had always taken great pride in his work.

(Here we see a clear pattern of repetition of domestic violence from one generation to the next. Perhaps the younger Albert was projecting his unresolved feelings about his mother onto his wife. Perhaps, too, a parallel could be drawn between Albert's diffidence about tracing his parentage in the past, and his avoidance of facing his cancer diagnosis now. Many terminally ill patients bring up some vivid recollection from long ago, and often this can be interpreted as having some link with their present situation.)

Della, seen alone, said 'I'm at the end of my tether.' She acknowledged that her marriage had not been happy. She had considered leaving Albert in the past, but was frightened of him, besides being financially dependent. Since becoming ill he had changed, wanting her to do everything for him, and stay with him all the time. At first, believing he would die very soon, she had resolved to do her best, giving in to his every whim and meekly keeping quiet when he shouted abuse. Now she felt unable to keep up this high standard of care, and longed to go out shopping or visiting friends, but dared not go 'because he makes me feel so guilty.'

(Albert is regressing to a child-like state in which he wants his wife to mother him, and take care of all his physical needs. He may be using his illness, whether deliberately or unconsciously, for secondary gain. Also, with his excessive demands and outbursts of abuse, he may be projecting his own unexpressed fear and anger about

continued

continued

what is happening to him. Della herself seems to be aspiring towards almost saintly behaviour and may be using the mechanism of sublimation to convert her past negative feelings into something quite opposite.)

It did not seem appropriate to embark on formal interpretive psychotherapy in this case. The longstanding nature of Albert's problems, his limited capacity for motivation and insight and his short life expectancy would not have made him a good candidate for such treatment. However, a brief and practical intervention did perhaps do some good. A joint meeting, including Albert, Della, a doctor and a nurse, began with a review of his physical condition, and a clear statement that his cancer was still progressing though at a very slow rate. Practical ways that Albert could receive the care he needed, and do the things he liked, while still allowing his wife and family a life of their own, were discussed. Albert's remark that he could no longer enjoy TV because 'there's so much violence and death' provided the interviewer with a ready opening for exploring his fear of dying, disguised as a fear of being left alone, and after this he broke down and cried. Della, clearly embarrassed, told him to pull himself together but he continued to weep. Afterwards he said it had done him a world of good.

A few weeks later, Albert developed another chest infection and, because of the difficulties of nursing him in an overcrowded council house, was admitted to the ward for what soon became evident would be terminal care. He seemed to derive great comfort from the close nursing attention, saying 'It's wonderful here—I'm getting stronger day by day.' (This frank denial, sometimes found at the very end of life, probably does no harm.) Della and the children were constantly at his bedside until he peacefully died.

FURTHER READING

Holland JC. Clinical course of cancer. In Holland JC, Rowland JH (eds) (1989) *Handbook of Psychooncology*. Oxford University Press: New York

Rowland JH. Developmental stage and adaptation: adult model. In Holland JC, Rowland JH (eds) (1989a) *Handbook of Psychooncology*. Oxford University Press: New York.

Rowland JH. Intrapersonal resources: coping. In Holland JC, Rowland JH (eds) (1989b) *Handbook of Psychooncology*. Oxford University Press: New York

3
Emotional Problems in Cancer Patients

The majority of cancer patients, with the help of the various 'coping strategies' already outlined, manage to come to terms with their illness in ways which work reasonably well for them. Some, however, are unable to achieve a satisfactory emotional adjustment. Instead, they develop reactions of a kind which increase their own mental suffering, impair their relationships with other people, and prevent them gaining optimum benefit from anticancer treatments.

This part of the book begins by considering the frequency and causes of emotional problems. The classification of such problems is not clearcut. Although anxiety, depression, denial, anger, suicidality, confusion and somatisation will each be separately described, it is common to find mixed syndromes in clinical practice.

General principles of prevention and management are mentioned here, but more detail about specialised treatment methods for emotional problems will be found in Chapter 7.

GENERAL PRINCIPLES REGARDING EMOTIONAL PROBLEMS (Massie and Holland 1989)

Psychiatric Diagnoses in Cancer Patient Populations

Not all of the emotional distress found in cancer patients can, or should, be labelled as 'psychiatric illness' and several of the common problems, for example excessive anger or denial, do not fit with formal classification systems for psychiatric disorders. Nevertheless, psychiatric disorders occur more frequently in cancer patients than in the general population, and it is important to recognise them as there may be specific treatment available.

Several large-scale research surveys, using standardised interviews and diagnostic criteria such as the American Psychiatric Association's 'DSM-III-R' (*Diagnostic and Statistical Manual of Mental Disorders*, third revision) have reported on the frequency of psychiatric disorder in large populations of cancer patients. The findings vary somewhat depending on the site and stage of cancer concerned, but can be roughly summarised as follows:

* No psychiatric disorder: 50%
* Adjustment reaction: 30%
* Formal psychiatric diagnosis: 20%

An important observation, which some people find surprising, is that about half the patients have no significant psychiatric symptoms at all.

About one-third can be classified as having 'adjustment reactions'. These usually take the form of anxiety and/or depression, but of a kind which is readily understandable as a reaction to the physical illness. Although adjustment reactions are not serious mental disorders, and although they usually get better of their own accord in time, they do produce significant extra suffering for a great many cancer patients. Humane and well-organised general clinical care could often do much to minimise this distress.

About one-fifth of patients have a formal psychiatric diagnosis. Again, depression and/or anxiety are the most common forms, but more severe and different in kind from the adjustment disorders, and meriting specialised treatment. The organic brain syndromes are also included here. So are the other psychiatric conditions—schizophrenia, affective psychoses, personality disorders, obsessive–compulsive disorders and eating disorders for example—which are no more common in cancer patients than in the general population, but on rare occasions coexist with cancer by chance. Such cases often present difficult management problems calling for psychiatric advice.

Causes of Emotional Problems

It is seldom possible to pinpoint with confidence any one precise cause in the individual patient, but one or more of the following factors often contribute:

- The psychological stresses of the cancer diagnosis, for example concern about future prognosis and about welfare of relatives.
- Poorly controlled physical symptoms: for example pain, nausea, breathlessness.
- A past history of psychiatric illness.
- A vulnerable personality, not good at coping with stress.
- Biological factors directly affecting the brain: primary or secondary cerebral tumours, metabolic disturbances such as liver failure, drug side-effects.
- Poor relationships with healthcare professionals: lack of communication, fear of being abandoned as the disease progresses.
- Lack of supportive confiding relationships with family and friends.
- Other life events and social difficulties not directly connected to the cancer, for example a recent bereavement.

Prevention of Emotional Problems

Emotional problems would be minimised if some basic principles of good clinical practice were more widely applied. The following guidelines apply to all healthcare professionals and do not require any specialised psychological skills.

- Offer information about the illness and its treatment: 'too little' information is a far more frequent complaint than 'too much'. Avoid needless delays in passing on new information to the patient. Remember that information given on one occasion is often forgotten or misinterpreted, and may need to be repeated later, or backed up with written material.
- Allow the patient to participate in treatment decisions, if he or she wishes to do so.

- Allow the patient to express emotional distress, making it clear there is no cause for shame in this. Many patients consider it weak or ungrateful to break down in tears, although they have ample reason to be upset and may well feel a great deal better for a good cry. The 'pull yourself together and keep a stiff upper lip' response shown by some relatives and professionals is not helpful.
- Provide ongoing care from a few key doctors and nurses who will be there to monitor both physical progress and emotional wellbeing throughout the course of the illness. The patient's own general practitioner should be one of these. In hospital settings, try to arrange continuity of care so the patient sees the same person at each clinic visit.

Detection of Emotional Problems

There is plenty of research evidence to show that emotional problems among cancer patients often go unrecognised unless they are specifically sought out, either through personal interviews or by means of a screening questionnaire such as the HAD (Hospital Anxiety and Depression) Scale. Because emotional problems can arise at any time during the course of an illness, such screening should ideally be repeated at regular intervals for each patient. Putting this apparently simple recommendation into practice requires consistent effort on behalf of the staff.

Whether or not a formal screening programme is in place, it is important that all patients are asked from time to time how they are coping with the emotional side of their illness, and given frequent opportunities to discuss their current concerns.

While emotional problems are still frequently missed, there is also a risk—especially as oncology staff become more sophisticated in psychological matters—of their being overdiagnosed. Symptoms with a significant biological basis, for example mood changes following increase or decrease of steroid dosage, may be interpreted as purely psychogenic reactions unless the close interdependence of 'physical' and 'mental' phenomena is recognised by oncologists and mental health professionals alike.

Management of Emotional Problems

The same points listed above under 'prevention' are also the first steps in 'management' when an emotional problem has already developed. A single interview in which the patient is given plenty of time to express feelings, ask questions and clear up any factual misunderstandings, with the promise of followup support, often brings striking benefit.

Before going on to more specific interventions, it is worth making a detached judgement of whether there really *is* an emotional problem present, and if so, whether it lies primarily with the patient rather than with relatives or staff. It is also worth reviewing the patient's physical status because organic brain syndromes are easily overlooked unless frank confusion is present.

'Specific interventions' include psychological techniques and psychotropic drugs. These are best delivered by an experienced mental health professional, but the criteria for deciding to refer will depend on what service is available locally. Having a named specialist who works, even part-time, as a member of the oncology team is usually preferable to calling in the duty psychiatrist from a separate unit. Referral to a mental health professional should be discussed openly with the patient beforehand. Some doctors and nurses avoid doing this, because of their own embarrassment about emotional topics, with the result that the consultation gets off to a bad start from which it may never recover.

Outcome of Emotional Problems

Emotional problems among cancer patients can get better. The outcome is naturally more hopeful for cases in which the cancer itself has a favourable prognosis, but even patients with advanced cancer can come through periods of distress and achieve emotional serenity at the end of their lives.

DEPRESSION (Cody 1990; Haig 1992; Massie 1989; Mermelstein and Lesko 1992)

Depression is among the most frequent of emotional problems in cancer patients, and is important because it can often be treated successfully. Surveys show that up to 50% of patients at any one time report some depressive symptoms, with 10-20% having a fullblown depressive illness. Depression is estimated to be four times more frequent in patients with cancer than in the population as a whole.

Depression in cancer patients can be difficult to diagnose, and is easily missed.

'Normal' and 'Pathological' Depression

Depressed mood is a frequent response to unpleasant life situations, especially those which involve a loss. Many cancer patients, though not all, go through a period of feeling depressed after first learning their diagnosis, or in reaction to disease progression or relapse. This is often an appropriate stage in the adjustment process, and some experts actually consider it a desirable one which will ultimately help to promote realistic acceptance. 'Sadness' would perhaps be a better term than 'depression '.

This appropriate normal reaction merges into the pathological form of depression (clinical depression; depressive illness) which is more severe and prolonged. Some patients report that the depressed mood found in this condition has a different quality from ordinary sadness. The lowered mood is accompanied by other characteristic symptoms as listed below.

Depression cannot always be put down simply to the psychological stress of having cancer. Some cancer patients are depressed in response to unrelated life events and difficulties, for example a bereavement or a marital problem. Some have a constitutional vulnerability to depression, as shown by a past history or family history of this condition. In others, biological complications of cancer—for example, hypercalcaemia or cerebral metastases—are contributing. Cancer of the pancreas appears to have a special association with depression, for reasons which are unknown. Side-effects of drugs, including cytotoxics and steroids, must also be considered. Usually, in any one patient, a mixture of several contributory factors is present.

Symptoms

Depression has both mental and physical symptoms.

Mental symptoms include low mood, characteristically worse in the mornings and lifting as the day goes on (diurnal variation), tearfulness (but sometimes an inability to cry), guilt, feeling a burden to other people, loss of interest, inability to feel pleasure (anhedonia), poor concentration, agitation or retardation, irritability, social withdrawal, and suicidal thoughts.

Physical symptoms include weight loss, anorexia, insomnia (characteristically with early morning waking), tiredness, malaise and pain. Because these same physical symptoms are often found in advanced cancer, they may not be very helpful in making a diagnosis of depression. Depression should be suspected, however, if the physical symptoms seem out of proportion to the stage of cancer progression.

Depression is often unrecognised because depressed patients are reluctant to complain about their symptoms; and because the most prominent symptom is not always the obvious one of low mood. Other presentations in cancer patients include anxiety, difficult-to-control pain, thoughts about suicide or euthanasia, or a lack of motivation and energy as observed by the staff. Patients who deny feeling low or depressed, but have other symptoms suggesting a depressive illness, may respond well to antidepressant drugs.

Clinical Types of Depression

Some psychiatrists favour classifying depressive illness into various types. The complexities involved are beyond the scope of this book, but it is appropriate to give a warning about the rather old-fashioned terms 'endogenous' and 'reactive' depression. These terms refer to two symptom clusters at the extreme ends of a spectrum, with most cases falling in the middle range. However, the terms are often misinterpreted as referring solely to the presumed *cause* of the depression, with the unfortunate result that depression in cancer patients is considered so obviously 'reactive' that nobody treats it seriously. The flaw in this viewpoint has often been illustrated by pointing out that nobody withholds analgesics from cancer patients because their pain has an understandable cause! When symptoms of clinical depression are present, whether or not the patient has good reason to be depressed, psychiatric assessment and treatment are worthwhile.

How Depression can Affect Cancer Treatment

Depressed patients may consider themselves too worthless to merit help; therefore they do not complain either about the symptoms of depression or those of their cancer. Physically they tend to look worse than they are, and the symptoms of the depression may be taken as evidence of tumour advancement. The end result of all these factors may be that investigations and treatment are given up prematurely.

Differential Diagnosis of Depression

The distinction from 'normal' sadness, and from physical deterioration, has been mentioned above and is one that even experienced psychiatrists can have great difficulty in making.

Biological complications of cancer such as hypercalcaemia and cerebral metastases, and prescribed drugs such as steroids and certain chemotherapeutic agents, may lead to depression in vulnerable people.

Other physical illnesses besides cancer can mimic depression; hypothyroidism is the classic example.

Management of Depression

Depressed or unhappy patients should first be offered an opportunity to express their feelings of sadness or anger about the losses of the illness and how unfair it all seems. Many patients benefit greatly from a sympathetic acknowledgement of their distress. This can often be achieved through just one or two long interviews, which will often include some tears as well as talking. Fostering a 'fighting spirit' in cancer patients is fashionable at present, partly because there is preliminary evidence linking this attitude to improved physical survival. The 'downside' of this trend is to accentuate the sense of shame and failure often felt by patients who are depressed. They need to know that depression is a perfectly acceptable response to having cancer, and that open expression of negative feelings about the illness—as opposed to bottling them up—can actually form part of the fighting spirit response. Some patients need to work through a depressive stage before they are able to muster a more positive outlook.

Many depressed cancer patients say they have not been given enough information about their diagnosis, treatment or prognosis. Whether information has been genuinely lacking, or whether patients themselves have been unable to take it in, this aspect may require attention.

If depression persists more than a few weeks, and does not respond to simple discussion of facts and ventilation of feelings, more specialised treatment in the form of psychotherapy and/or antidepressant drugs will be required. An ongoing relationship with one or more trusted doctors and nurses remains essential alongside such treatments.

A successful outcome of depression in advanced cancer is illustrated by the following case history.

Donald (44) had cancer of the prostate, with widespread bony metastases already present on diagnosis. He had received radiotherapy and hormonal treatment. His mood was low 'on and off' and he commented that the pain in his back seemed much worse when he felt depressed. His sleep was disturbed, without any fixed pattern. His main concerns were the forced inactivity, for he had been an active man who loved hill-walking, and the prospect of separation from his wife when he died. He cried throughout the psychiatric assessment interview and appeared sunk in despair.

Treatment with amitriptyline was combined with regular discussions in which he raised such issues as his wish to die in hospital rather than at home, and his reactions to witnessing the death of another patient in the opposite bed. He was also encouraged to set practical short-term goals, for example spending a weekend at home.

The amitriptyline was increased to the upper limit of his tolerance which proved to be 200 mg at night, a higher dose than usually given in palliative care settings. His mood showed a striking improvement, which he attributed not so much to the drug as to the opportunity to unburden his distress during the assessment interview— 'Before then I'd bottled it up, like stoking a fire that won't burn.' He remained in good spirits for the remaining two weeks of his life.

ANXIETY (Maguire, Faulkner and Regnard 1993; Massie 1989)

Anxiety and depression are often mixed in the same patient.

'Normal' and 'Pathological' Anxiety

Almost everyone is familiar with the emotion called anxiety. Most people feel anxious in a situation which is unfamiliar, uncertain or frankly dangerous. Some degree of anxiety among patients with cancer is therefore understandable and does not require psychiatric labels or treatments.

Around the time of initial diagnosis, most though not all patients feel anxiety. Paradoxical as it may seem, many express relief when the diagnosis of cancer is confirmed—knowing the truth is easier than fearing the unknown. As the illness progresses, anxiety may be rekindled by further points of uncertainty—waiting to begin a new treatment, being admitted to hospital for the first time, waiting for the results of diagnostic tests for suspected relapse.

Some patients suffer more anxiety than they need at such times, because they are harbouring ungrounded fears about their illness or its treatment and are too frightened to mention these to the staff looking after them. Accurate factual information may dispel such fears. At the opposite extreme, some anxious patients seek out more information than they can cope with, for example reading up possible side-effects of the proposed treatment and worrying they will develop them all.

When anxiety develops for no apparent reason, or persists in a disabling form long after its initial cause has passed, an 'anxiety disorder' may be diagnosed. This happens for some cancer patients who remain disabled by anxiety about their illness even if from a physical point of view they appear to be doing well.

Symptoms

Anxiety is accompanied by both mental (psychological) and physical (somatic) symptoms. Many anxious patients have a combination of mental and physical symptoms, each exacerbating the other so that a vicious circle develops. Mental symptoms are usually quite easy to recognise: worry, irritability, restlessness, difficulty in getting off to sleep or sleep disturbed by nightmares.

Physical symptoms, most of which can be explained by overbreathing, overactivity of the autonomic nervous system or muscle tension, may affect any body system and lead to diagnostic difficulties because neither doctor nor patient suspects an emotional cause. Common symptoms of this kind include breathlessness, palpitations, sweating, headaches, a 'lump in the throat' which impedes swallowing, nausea, abdominal pain and diarrhoea.

Clinical Types of Anxiety

Anxiety may be present continuously most of the time, or in acute bouts (*panic attacks*). A distinction can often be made between *trait* anxiety, which has been present throughout life as an integral feature of the personality, and *state* anxiety which has arisen anew in reaction to stressful circumstances. *Phobic anxiety* is that provoked by a specific stimulus, common examples in cancer patients being intravenous injections, or being left alone in a radiation chamber. Other patients suffer from *generalised* or *free-floating* anxiety which they cannot relate to any particular cause, though in someone with cancer it is often a reasonable supposition that such anxiety is due to unexpressed fear of progressive disease and of death. Fear of being alone at night-time is a common presentation of this.

How Anxiety can Affect Cancer Treatment

Some chronically anxious patients have a very low threshold for consulting a doctor. Diagnosis of cancer in such patients is sometimes delayed because they have 'cried wolf' so often before. After cancer has actually been confirmed, they may become increasingly hypochondriacal. Concern about treatment side-effects, and false alarms about spread of the disease, are likely to be common. At the opposite extreme, anxious patients may be so frightened of cancer that they keep their symptoms a secret, so that diagnosis is long delayed. Phobic anxiety may interfere with diagnostic tests or the delivery of treatment.

Differential Diagnosis of Anxiety

Especially in patients who are acutely physically ill, biological conditions which mimic anxiety should be considered. These include uncontrolled pain, metabolic disorders such as hypoxia and hypoglycaemia, internal haemorrhage, drugs (steroids can cause anxiety; neuroleptics can cause the mental and physical restlessness known as akathisia), and drug withdrawal (alcohol, benzodiazepines). Hormone-secreting tumours are a rare cause, and thyrotoxicosis can cause symptoms identical to those of anxiety.

Management of Anxiety

Anxiety can be minimised by the sympathetic organisation of treatment services, for example letting patients know the results of tests as soon as these come through, rather than making them wait days or weeks for their next outpatient visit; providing continuity of care from familiar doctors and nurses; and trying to give the right amount of information, neither too little nor too much, in each individual case.

Explaining the origin of physical symptoms may help, for example headaches may become much less troublesome if the patient can be convinced they are due to muscle tension rather than a brain tumour. Physical treatments like massage and relaxation may be specially helpful when physical symptoms are prominent.

Behavioural (relaxation, distraction, hypnosis, desensitisation) and cognitive techniques are most useful for phobic anxiety. Drugs used for anxiety include benzodiazepines, antidepressants and beta-blockers.

The following case illustrates the common combination of anxiety with depression.

Raymond, a 45-year-old married medical records clerk, developed bleeding from a mole on his cheek which was excised and found to be a malignant melanoma. A few months later, metastases developed in his liver and lungs, and he began a course of cytotoxic chemotherapy. A psychiatric referral was made because he seemed both anxious and depressed.

He described panic attacks in relation to medical procedures, specifically blood tests or intravenous injections, and being confined under X-ray machines. He also described a 'morbid fascination' with melanoma, leading him to read the notes of other cases at work although he realised that 'a little knowledge is a dangerous thing '. He revealed some questions which were troubling him, for example whether chemotherapy given earlier on would have prevented metastases from developing. He had not put his questions to the oncologist 'in case I don't like the answers '. He had always been rather an anxious man, and had had two episodes of depression in early adult life.

Following a general discussion of his fears, Raymond's therapy included a combination of techniques. He was encouraged to write down and rehearse the questions he wanted to ask his consultant; to go and see the MRI scanner a few days before he was to be scanned; and to begin a structured programme of activities in his leisure time, including some (bird-watching, going to the cinema) which he and his wife had enjoyed before his illness but lately not bothered to pursue. A tricyclic antidepressant was prescribed to help his sleep and lift his mood. Although his physical disease continued to progress, Raymond's mental adjustment improved considerably.

DENIAL (Greer 1992)

The Concept of Denial

Denial, perhaps the best-known of the 'ego defence mechanisms', involves an unconscious refusal to acknowledge certain distressing aspects of reality. Most people use denial to protect themselves against anxiety and unpleasantness in daily life—they 'turn a blind eye' to things they prefer not to know about. Those who forget to pay the gas bill or visit the dentist, who consider themselves to be perfectly happily married until their partners leave home, or who continue to flout medical warnings against heavy smoking and drinking, may be using denial.

No objective method of measuring denial exists; its presence can only be inferred from the judgement of other people. Devising a valid questionnaire to measure denial is probably impossible, though some attempts have been made.

The term 'denial' is often used in relation to cancer patients who apparently fail to realise their diagnosis or the gravity of their prognosis. Denial may be suspected when the patient fails to ask any questions about the illness despite ample opportunity; 'forgets' the information given; makes unrealistic plans for the future; or seems to understand matters in an intellectual sense without showing appropriate emotional distress. Patients who are older and less well educated are probably most likely to show denial, but striking exceptions may occur.

Barclay, an ambitious young lawyer, had cancer of the colon with liver metastases. He read up the technical aspects of his illness in great detail and asked many questions about his chemotherapy treatment. He never appeared anything but cheerful and optimistic, and steadfastly continued to claim that he was going to make a full recovery, despite obviously deepening jaundice and marked loss of weight. This stance came over so forcefully that neither his wife nor the staff looking after him felt able to question it. He died without making a will, and having just posted off an application for career promotion. Afterwards, although his wife was sad that she had been unable to talk with him more fully, she felt that his attitude had been in keeping with his personality and enabled him to enjoy life to the end.

Such complete and sustained denial is rare, but partial and fluctuating denial is common. Depending on the degree of denial, and the circumstances in which it occurs, denial may be either a healthy psychological defence mechanism (adaptive denial) or a source of problems for the patient and others (maladaptive denial). Sometimes, as in the case described above, its effects are a mixture of both good and bad.

Adaptive Denial

A temporary period of denial often follows the initial diagnosis of cancer or of a first recurrence. Many patients would be overwhelmed by facing up to the full implications of such bad news all at once, whereas letting it sink in gradually is more bearable. Denial may also be observed in patients who are dying. Transient denial at such crisis points in the illness is a natural means of emotional self-protection.

In the longer term, lesser degrees of denial merge with the strategy of 'looking on the bright side' (in more technical language, 'positive appraisal'). Dying patients who daydream about next summer's holiday without actually making a booking are using a harmless fantasy to maintain hope. Patients whose psychological make-up enables them to use denial in this way can often be considered fortunate; they are less vulnerable to depression and anxiety than those who appreciate the grim realities of their condition more starkly. Sometimes, however, their defences get cruelly sabotaged by over-earnest staff who believe that all cancer patients must be made to face up to the truth.

Partial denial enables patients to acknowledge their cancer and accept the necessary treatment at one level of conscious awareness. At another level they play down the seriousness of the illness. One woman awaiting breast biopsy said 'My husband died from cancer so I know what it's all about, though in my case I'm confident there's nothing like that, it's only strain from heavy lifting.' A man attending a radiotherapy department remarked 'I suppose it's mainly cancer cases here' but claimed to have been told nothing about his own diagnosis. A young woman dying from ovarian cancer showed insight into her own denial when she said 'I certainly don't expect to expire for a very long time yet, but I'm not silly—I do accept I've got terminal cancer. It seems like two very strange ideas together. One half of me says I'm definitely going to die of cancer and the other says I'm definitely going to get better. '

Maladaptive Denial

More extreme and sustained forms of denial are undesirable because they may lead to delays in cancer diagnosis, poor compliance with treatment, blocked communication with relatives, and a failure to put one's practical affairs in order prior to death.

Women who ignore cancerous lumps in the breast until they become fixed and ulcerating may be using denial, as suggested by such comments as:

'I didn't take much notice. '

'I don't believe in searching for nasties. '

'I thought everyone had lumps like this. '

Sometimes, too, complete denial suddenly breaks down towards the end of life to expose overwhelming distress.

Differential Diagnosis of Denial

Denial was originally described in psychoanalytic theory as an unconscious phenomenon. However, it can be impossible to distinguish this from a deliberate strategy. Many patients are in fact well aware of the truth about their illness but prefer not to think or talk about it: 'cognitive avoidance' or 'suppression '. One elderly man always euphemistically referred to his bowel cancer as 'the main problem' and said 'It's best not to burden myself or others by discussing it, although I admit it lurks in the background like a big black cloud.' He politely declined all opportunites to talk in greater depth, but appeared to make a reasonably contented adjustment to his situation all the same.

Other patients, usually those who are not very intelligent or well educated, are exhibiting *ignorance* rather than denial. Some might welcome a frank explanation of their illness, but are inhibited from asking anybody, either because they are too much in awe of doctors and nurses as authority figures, or because they are so unfamiliar with medical terminology that they neither know how to phrase their questions nor would be likely to understand the answers.

Organic brain syndromes may be associated with somewhat bizarre variants of denial.

Robin, a man in his late 20s who had an inoperable brain tumour, usually maintained a bland cheery air. He showed no concern about his illness, nor about his many social problems which included heavy debts and a broken marriage. Then, following a sudden deterioration of his physical condition—he had developed weakness of both legs—he asked a nurse for euthanasia. Further exploration of this request revealed his fear of becoming paralysed and blind, and dread of being a burden to others. These concerns seemed appropriate, and psychiatric assessment revealed no symptoms of clinical depression. He agreed to continued discussions with the psychiatrist, which took place every few days. During some of these sessions the content of his talk was quite rational and his mood appropriately sad. At other times he appeared, as before, perfectly cheerful; on one occasion he stated that his only worry was where to buy some bright red Christmas wrapping paper, and on another that he intended to train as a doctor when his health improved.

In this case, as in many others, the denial was probably not harming the patient and to challenge it could be cruel.

Denial in Relation to Prognosis of Cancer

Some research suggests that denial predicts a good physical prognosis in patients with early breast cancer. This intriguing finding requires confirmation in further studies.

Management of Denial

Staff may adopt one of two extreme approaches with patients who are showing denial: collusion and confrontation.

Collusion involves going along with the patient's self-deception, pretending that there is indeed nothing much wrong and that everything is going to be alright. This is often the easiest line to take, and for some patients is indeed the kindest, but many staff feel uncomfortable with it. The opposite approach is *confrontation*—challenging the patient with the truth. Either of these two extremes may be right in some circumstances, but collusion may leave those involved feeling dissatisfied, whereas confrontation is all too often undertaken mainly for the benefit of staff themselves, and risks provoking great distress in the patient.

How different staff members choose to handle denial depends very much on their own personalities, and their intuitive feel for the patient concerned. My own view is that a middle course is best: giving patients ample opportunity to question the situation but never forcing unwanted information upon them.

During the 1970s and 1980s, when the old-fashioned secrecy about cancer was being swept away, 'denial' tended to be used as a term of criticism for patients who lacked the moral fibre to face up to their diagnosis. The 1990s view is more tolerant, for denial is now recognised as a valuable coping mechanism, which most people probably use at one time or another. Unless there is some compelling reason to interfere, patients should not be denied the use of denial.

ANGER (Faulkner, Maguire and Regnard 1994)

Transient anger after receiving a diagnosis of cancer is described as a normal phase in the adjustment process. Some patients can obtain a welcome release through spontaneous free expression of their anger, and then become able to move on towards emotional acceptance. In other patients anger becomes persistently ingrained, in which case it usually has destructive consequences for all concerned.

Jean, aged 60 and suffering from advanced ovarian cancer, was perceived as a 'difficult' patient on the ward where she was receiving palliative chemotherapy, having relapsed soon after her previous treatments with surgery and radiotherapy. The nursing staff felt she was silently critical towards them, and could not seem to build a rapport with her.

During psychiatric assessment she admitted having felt 'bottled up with anger inside' ever since the original diagnosis two years

continued

continued

previously, saying 'why should this happen to me?' and resentful of others' good health. She knew there was no rational target for this anger: 'It's nobody's fault, you can't find any reason' and 'I'm not the type to throw things.' She claimed that the doctors had led her to expect a complete cure from each of the previous treatments and felt 'everything's against me' when one treatment after the other had failed. She said 'I still live in hope' and expressed a wish for more information, but also admitted she did not want to hear any news that was not good. In her past history, she had been a fit active woman but admitted to having felt angry about other negative events including a broken marriage and some thwarted career ambitions.

At interview, she appeared very tense and angry but determined to remain in control of her feelings, clenching her teeth and fighting back the tears. She said the interview had made no difference to the way she felt, and declined any psychiatric followup.

Anger is sometimes more marked in relatives than patients themselves, as in the following case where it is mixed with denial.

Penelope, a divorcee in her 50s, lived with her 25-year-old son Martin, who suffered from an inoperable brain tumour. When he became unable to walk or talk, Penelope would not agree to his going into hospital, saying she wanted to nurse him back to health at home. Martin was a heavy man requiring constant care, but it was only with great reluctance that Penelope agreed to accept visits from district nurse, Macmillan nurse or care assistant. More often than not she would turn these professionals away when they called, saying they had chosen an inconvenient time, and sometimes reducing them to tears with her rudeness. Nobody could persuade her to acknowledge the seriousness of Martin's condition or talk about her own feelings. A few days before Martin died, when he was vomiting continually, a nurse found her trying to force a three-course home-cooked dinner into his mouth with a spoon. After his death, she wrote to accuse the hospital of killing him by negligence. Several independent experts agreed there had been no objective shortcomings in Martin's care.

Types of Anger

Anger may be:

- 'Free-floating,' when the patient is angry about the unfairness of the illness, perhaps blaming Fate or God.
- Displaced, often towards healthcare staff (this involves the mental mechanism of 'projection ').
- Justified, for example when there has been a delay in making the diagnosis or when treatment has caused more harm than good.
- Suppressed, so the patient does not acknowledge being angry and indeed may not be consciously aware of being so, but expresses the feeling indirectly; appearing negative and lacking cooperation, becoming depressed, developing somatic symptoms.

Management of Anger

Listen to the patient's point of view, without responding in a defensive fashion; and, however ungrateful and unrewarding the patient may seem to be, try to offer consistent professional concern. It may pay off in the end.

Providing time and space to facilitate full-blown expression of the anger—shouting, screaming, tears—may be cathartic and is best guided by a person with counselling skills who is not part of the physical care-giving team.

Giving clear and honest information about the illness should include acknowledging liability for any genuine shortcomings in care. Responding to criticisms of other doctors and nurses requires tact and skill. Colluding with putting the blame on colleagues is often both unwise and unfair—one usually only has the patient's side of the story. However, it is also inadvisable to make excuses for obvious mistakes. Often it is best just to listen without making judgements either way.

It may be appropriate to encourage redirection of anger, for example when a married couple seem to be taking out on each other their shared anger about the illness. Re-channelling energy elsewhere, towards for example exercise, music, creative activity or cancer-related charities, is sometimes an excellent strategy.

Psychotropic drugs (if the patient agrees to try them) may help if the anger is part of a psychiatric illness of depressive or paranoid type.

Entrenched anger often fails to respond to any of these interventions, as illustrated by the two case histories above.

SUICIDE AND SELF-HARM: VOLUNTARY EUTHANASIA

These topics overlap to some degree.

Suicide (Breitbart 1989)

Many physically healthy people believe that committing suicide would be the logical response to having cancer. In practice, few cancer patients react this way. One man told me 'It's funny, I always swore I'd shoot myself if I got the Big C, but now it's happened I don't mind at all. '

Many patients do admit they have thought about suicide. Knowing they have the option of ending their own lives, if and when their symptoms should become intolerable or they consider themselves too great a burden on their families, gives a sense of control over their future. Few of them actually take practical steps towards this end, and there is some evidence that suicidal thoughts and behaviour diminish as the cancer process advances. Perhaps, with modern palliative care, the terminal stage is not so bad as patients feared it was going to be; perhaps most terminal patients lack the energy or the practical means to kill themselves; or perhaps the instinct to live reasserts itself as natural death comes near.

Epidemiological studies indicate the suicide rate in patients with cancer is about twice that of the general population, and highest in the year after cancer diagnosis. However, official statistics probably understate the true frequency of suicide among patients with more advanced disease. Fatal overdose of sedatives or analgesics in such patients may go undetected; or the doctor may decide not to pursue the question of suicide which is in any doubt, in order to spare relatives the stigma and red tape resulting from police inquiries, a coroner's inquest and newspaper reports.

The excess of suicide among cancer patients is presumably due to the dread inspired by a cancer diagnosis, and/or the distressing symptoms of the disease. The same risk factors associated with suicide in the general population may also contribute. These include depressive illness, a past history of psychiatric disorder and/or previous suicide attempts, heavy drinking, and absence of supportive personal relationships. *Hopelessness* is believed to be a key theme underlying suicidal thoughts and behaviour.

While some cases of suicide among patients with cancer may be generally viewed as both understandable and justified, others represent the tragic culmination of distress which might have been relieved. The observations that several of the risk factors for suicide are potentially reversible, that many suicides have been in regular contact with healthcare professionals shortly before death, and that many have spoken about their intentions beforehand, all suggest that many such tragedies are preventable.

When suspicion of suicide risk is present, this should be tactfully explored with the patient. Suitable questions to introduce the topic might be 'How do you see the future?' 'Does it ever seem it's not worthwhile going on any longer?' or 'Have you considered harming yourself in any way?' Depending on the patient's response, more specific inquiries may follow, to see whether any practical action such as storing up medication has been planned or actually taken. Those firmly set on suicide may, of course, firmly deny their intentions, but many patients will be quite ambivalent about the matter and therefore glad of the opportunity to talk it over with a sympathetic person. Knowing that suicide would distress their relatives, or offend their own religious or moral code, they are willing to explore alternative solutions to their problems, and cooperate in preventive measures—for example letting somebody else look after their tablets, or accepting close observation from a companion or nurse.

Non-fatal Self-harm

Deliberate self-harm without a fatal outcome does not always represent a failed suicide attempt, as implied by some experts' use of the term 'parasuicide' in preference to 'attempted suicide '. Among young healthy members of the general population, many such acts can be seen as a 'cry for help' rather than a serious bid for self-destruction. Parasuicides are, however, at high risk of actually killing themselves eventually. Non-fatal self-harm by a cancer patient should certainly be taken seriously.

Oliver, a divorced man aged 67, refused chemotherapy after being diagnosed with lung cancer, saying 'I'm old and all alone, without an aim in life.' A few months later, while at home one weekend, he took a whole bottle of pain-killing tablets with some brandy. This made him sleep for several hours. He told a nurse about this overdose when attending hospital outpatients the following week, and a psychiatric assessment was arranged.

Oliver claimed he had seriously intended to end his life. His oncology casenotes contained reference to previous hints about suicide, and he had told one doctor 'If you won't put me down I'll do it myself.' He gave three reasons for his wish to die:

- Increasing chest pain, poorly controlled by medication (including the antidepressant drug amitriptyline, which he was taking in a dose of 100 mg at night).
- Loss of dignity; having valued privacy and independence all his life, he could not tolerate the prospect of needing help with personal selfcare, or being admitted to an institution.
- Loneliness; he lived alone, with no close relatives or friends, and had lost all social contacts since his retirement a few years earlier. The family doctor who knew him well had moved away the day before the overdose.

Oliver denied any previous suicide attempts, but it was later discovered that he had overdosed several times in the past.

The only evidence of a depressive illness was sleep disturbance with early morning waking, already improved by amitriptyline. The dose of this drug was gradually increased to 250 mg at night. Extra social support was arranged in the form of hospice Day Centre attendance and a volunteer to visit Oliver's home at weekends. A radiotherapy referral was made in respect of his chest pain.

Oliver grudgingly accepted these various forms of help. His sleep improved with the increase in amitriptyline. He lived another year, and his suicidal thoughts did not recur.

Overdose of drugs is the obvious means of suicide and self-harm for cancer patients. Other kinds of self-damaging behaviour such as non-compliance with medication, alcohol abuse or reckless driving may be indirect expressions of suicidal ideas, as may requests for euthanasia.

Voluntary Euthanasia (Saunders 1992)

Voluntary euthanasia—deliberately ending the life of a patient with incurable illness, at the patient's own request—is illegal, although current debate on the issue may well lead to a change in the law in certain parts of the world.

Euthanasia should be distinguished from two other medical practices which have long been considered acceptable. One is administration of adequate doses of pain-relieving drugs which may incidentally have the effect of shortening life. The other is the withholding, or withdrawal, of specific treatment which might have prolonged life but does not appear to be in the patient's best interests. Especially in the USA, 'advance directives' or 'living wills' are being introduced, so that patients can make their wishes about withdrawal of treatment known beforehand. Some requests for euthanasia represent pleas for better control of pain or other symptoms, better communication, relief for relatives to whom the patient feels a burden, or signal the presence of clinical depression.

Granting this request for euthanasia, without a clinical trial of antidepressant treatment and social support, would have

Kate, age 77, a retired headmistress of robust previous personality, had metastatic breast cancer causing breathlessness and back-ache. She felt 'devastated—I always thought my husband would die first—I'd rather try something like Exit than put my family through this ordeal.' ('Exit' was a former name for the Voluntary Euthanasia Society.) Whenever she thought about her illness, she suffered attacks of panic with tight breathing and a racing heart. She felt low in mood and could only maintain interest and concentration for a short time. A few days later Kate had taken to bed and was continually demanding euthanasia. She spoke en-viously of a friend who had recently committed suicide, saying 'That would be much the best in my case.' Asked how her family might react, she replied casually, 'Oh, they'd soon get over it.'

continued

continued

> A provisional diagnosis of depression was made, and amitriptyline commenced in a dose of 25 mg at night, gradually increased to 75 mg. Support was organised in the form of Day Centre attendance, with home visits from a Macmillan nurse in between.
> Within a week she was transformed, out of bed and cooking meals, and requesting a blood transfusion 'to give a further boost'. She remained in a cheerful, mentally alert state, enjoying frequent visits from her family and friends, and made no further mention of euthanasia during the remaining six months of her life.

deprived Kate herself of what proved to be several months of worthwhile living, and almost certainly would have left her husband and daughters with more distressing memories in their bereavement. It must be accepted, however, that not all case histories have such a satisfactory ending as Kate's.

Many doctors are against euthanasia because they fear it would soon become 'voluntary' only in name. Patients might feel obliged to request it, regarding themselves as a nuisance or burden to their relatives or to the state. Frail or confused patients incapable of making their own informed choice might be disposed of to suit the convenience of other people, or to save money. The inevitable changes in professional attitudes which would follow introduction of euthanasia would conflict with the present life-enhancing philosophy of medicine and nursing. Some claim that euthanasia requests would never arise if all patients with incurable illness received the benefits of skilled palliative care.

If euthanasia were to be legalised, its practice would need to be carefully regulated to guard against abuse, and ensure it was never carried out until every effort had been made to relieve pain, depression, social isolation and professional neglect.

ORGANIC BRAIN SYNDROMES: CONFUSION AND ACUTE DISTURBANCE (Fleishman and Lesko 1989; Stedeford 1987; Stedeford and Regnard 1991)

Various physical (organic, biological) complications of cancer and its treatment can disturb the functioning of the brain. The usual clinical presentation, in everyday language, is one of *confusion*.

Acute cases of severe agitated confusion arise from time to time on cancer treatment wards, creating a combined medical and psychiatric emergency. Milder cases are much more common, especially among older patients and those whose general physical condition is poor; these are often missed.

A simplified classification of confusion distinguishes two main clinical syndromes: *delirium* and *dementia*. Delirium, or *acute organic brain syndrome*, is potentially reversible whereas dementia, or *chronic organic brain syndrome*, usually involves a permanent impairment of brain function. Elements of both syndromes often exist together in the same patient.

Some patients who superficially appear to be confused do not really have either of these syndromes. In elderly patients who are anxious about being ill and coming into the strange environment of a hospital, against a background of slight deafness or forgetfulness, apparent 'confusion' will often settle down after they have been given careful repeated explanations of where they are and what is happening.

On some wards, all new patients are asked to complete a simple test of cognitive function, for example the MiniMental State, as part of the admission routine. Such a screening procedure will pick up cases of mild confusion which were not obvious otherwise, and also provide a baseline score if florid confusion develops later on.

The major part of this chapter will be devoted to delirium. Although dementia occasionally develops as a direct complication of cancer, notably in brain tumour patients, most dementias result from a separate pathological process such as Alzheimer's disease, and coexist with the cancer only by chance.

Delirium can be briefly defined as follows:

'Clouding of consciousness, accompanied by changes in perception, thought and mood, from an organic cause. '

Clinical Features

Presenting symptoms of delirium might include getting lost on the ward; putting on clothes the wrong way round; misidentifying people or places; behaviour which is sexually disinhibited (groping at women, walking around naked) or dangerous (wandering outside the ward, smoking in bed); becoming irritable, suspicious (paranoid) or withdrawn; saying things which do not make sense. Past memories may seem to be mixed up with present experiences, and bodily sensations mistaken for perceptions of the surrounding environment. Symptoms develop within a few hours or days, and may fluctuate over short periods of time. Many patients have altered sleep patterns, and become more confused at night.

The headings of the *Mental State Examination* can be used to organise a description of the patient's condition, as follows:

- *Appearance and behaviour*—does the patient look ill? Any abnormal movements? Able to cooperate with the interview?
- *Talk*—spontaneous or only in answer to questions? Coherent? Write down a few word-for-word examples of any unusual statements.
- *Mood*—depressed, anxious, euphoric, frightened, suspicious, labile? Anxiety and confusion can each exacerbate the other to form a vicious circle.
- *Thought content*—this may give useful clues to patient's underlying concerns, as discussed below.
- *Abnormal beliefs and experiences*—misperceptions (faulty interpretations of real stimuli, for example mistaking voices on the radio for staff discussing the patient), hallucinations (false perceptions such as seeing animals in the bed), and delusions (false beliefs such as 'this place is not a hospital ').
- *Cognitive function*—orientation (in time, place and person), attention and concentration (serial subtraction of 7 from 100, to make 93, 86, 79 etc; listing the months of the year backwards), long- and short-term memory, general information, current affairs.
- *Insight*—is the patient aware of being confused?

Causes of Delirium

The majority of delirious patients have more than one disorder which could be contributing to their confusion. Examples of the many different possible causes are listed below. Some affect the brain directly, whereas others are systemic. Not all of them are due to the cancer. Some are 'iatrogenic ', the result of medical intervention.

- Drugs: opioids, psychotropics, steroids, anticholinergics ('hot as a hare, blind as a bat, dry as a bone, red as a beet, mad as a hatter ').
- Drug withdrawal: opioids, benzodiazepines, alcohol.
- Infections: chest, urinary.
- Organ failure: cardiac, respiratory, renal, hepatic.
- Biochemical disturbance: hypercalcaemia.
- Cerebral lesions: primary or secondary brain tumour, stroke.

Assessing the Confused Patient

A detailed *history* is desirable, but it will be impossible to obtain this from the patient. Relatives, and old casenotes, can often give useful background information. Previous similar episodes may, for example, have resolved after treatment of a urinary infection or of hypercalcaemia. A history of forgetfulness or 'personality change' going back several months or years may suggest underlying dementia.

Review the *drug chart*. Was anything new prescribed shortly before the onset of the confusion? Consider tapering off any drugs of doubtful value. Also consider a drug withdrawal syndrome—have opioids or benzodiazepines recently been reduced or discontinued? Alcohol withdrawal syndrome (delirium tremens) may develop when patients who were drinking heavily at home are suddenly deprived of alcohol in hospital.

Physical examination may show, for example, signs of infection or raised intracranial pressure. The choice of *laboratory investigations* should be guided by the findings on history and examination. An investigation is seldom justified unless its result would alter the clinical management. Blood count, urea and electrolytes, serum calcium, liver function tests, midstream urine specimen and chest X-ray will often be relevant. More specialised tests, such as a brain scan, should be considered if there are specific clinical indications.

Medical review should be carried out frequently—several times daily in severe cases—and the findings recorded in the casenotes.

Prompt detection, investigation and treatment of delirium is important. A patient who is becoming slightly muddled may not attract top priority on a busy ward. If nothing is done, however, the patient may present an acutely disturbed or even violent state in the middle of the night; and by the time that stage is reached, the chances of successful treatment are not so good.

The symptomatic management of confusion is discussed below under three headings: practical, psychological and pharmacological. Drug treatment is deliberately considered last—it is not good practice to rush into giving tranquillisers, although many doctors and nurses automatically respond to a confused patient in this way.

Practical Management

Unfamiliar people and places can worsen a patient's confusion, so keep changes of nursing staff to the minimum, do not allow too many visitors, and try to keep the patient in the same bed, unless a move is essential to avoid such hazards as high windows and unguarded ward exits. Frank physical restraint, such as confinement to a locked room, should be avoided if at all possible.

Familiar people and places can help. Try to organise constant observation and support from a small team of known and trusted staff. Keep the room well-lit, and consider bringing in some 'orienting objects ', such as a clock or photos of the family from the patient's home. Beware, however, of objects which could be dangerous, such as matches or a glass vase. Ensure the patient is comfortable: wet sheets, crumbs in the bed, and noisy surroundings may be adding to the confusion.

Psychological Management

Most confused patients feel bewildered and afraid. Medical and nursing procedures may frighten them even more. They should always be given a careful explanation before anything is done to them (blood taken, sheets changed), even if they do not appear to understand what they are told.

Formal psychotherapy for patients with organic brain dysfunction obviously has marked limitations. It is both pointless and cruel to press psychological concepts on a patient who is too ill to understand them. There is also a danger that pursuing a psychotherapeutic approach will divert attention from the medical disorder which needs treatment. However, there are times when a simple psychological interpretation can help to make sense of apparently bizarre experiences and reveal important aspects of the patients' concerns. A patient who mistakes his doctor for a policeman, for example, might perhaps be feeling guilty about some misdeed from his own past; alternatively, such a mistake might imply something about the personality of the doctor concerned! Gently exploring the content of confused patients' speech or behaviour may enable them to admit for the first time what is really worrying them, and perhaps become less confused.

The relatives should be kept well-informed. The fear and stigma commonly associated with 'going mad' can sometimes be reduced by pointing out that the physical illness, rather than the patient's true self, is responsible for the strange behaviour.

Drug Treatment

In theory, confusion is best managed by treating its cause(s), rather than adding extra medication which might complicate matters further. In practice, however, sedation is often required to treat patients' agitation and distress, and reduce the risk of harm to themselves or others. Many patients who are otherwise suspicious of medication will accept a night-time dose of 'something to help with sleep'.

Oral medication should be used if possible. Liquid formulations may be accepted more readily than tablets. An injection may be necessary if the patient is too ill to take the drug by mouth, and in emergencies.

Neuroleptics (antipsychotic drugs) quieten disturbed patients without causing impairment of consciousness, and control 'psychotic' symptoms such as delusions and hallucinations.

Haloperidol, which can be given orally, intramuscularly, subcutaneously or intravenously, is a suitable choice. Starting dose is usually 5 mg, though smaller doses (1.5 or 3 mg) may be preferred for the elderly or frail. Alternative drugs include *chlorpromazine* and *thioridazine.* In an emergency the dose can be repeated at hourly or half-hourly intervals until sedation is achieved. Short-term adverse effects include hypotension, and extrapyramidal symptoms such as torticollis (twisting of the neck). Extrapyramidal symptoms can be controlled by an anticholinergic drug such as *procyclidine* 5–10 mg by the oral, intramuscular or intravenous route.

Benzodiazepines are an alternative to the neuroleptics. Examples are *diazepam* 10–40 mg given orally, intravenously, intramuscularly or rectally; *lorazepam* 1–5 mg either intramuscularly, intravenously or sublingually; and *midazolam,* which given by slow subcutaneous infusion is popular for treating agitation in the terminally ill.

Barbiturates are occasionally used when other drugs have failed.

Combinations of two drugs from different groups, for example haloperidol and diazepam, may be required but single-drug therapy should be tried first.

If drugs are to be used at all, they should be given in adequate dosage. By all means begin with small amounts for patients whose general condition is poor, but do not be afraid to go higher if need be.

Compulsory Treatment

Application of the Mental Health Act (1983) is occasionally required for patients who present a danger to themselves or others but are refusing to stay in hospital or accept treatment.

This legislation only applies to patients suffering from mental disorder, including mental disorder which is secondary to physical disorder. Seek advice from a psychiatrist, or a social worker approved under the Act, or a medical defence society. If in doubt, emergency treatment in the patient's best interests may be given under common law.

In many clinical situations relevant to oncology, application of the Mental Health Act is not appropriate. It could not, for example, be used to enforce anticancer treatment for patients who do not want it, or to detain patients whose relatives do not want them home.

Outcome of Delirium

Depending on the severity of the condition, and the nature of the underlying pathology, the outcome of delirium may be:

- Complete recovery.
- Survival with residual dementia.
- Progression to coma and death.

The likelihood of a good outcome is improved if the clinical symptoms are picked up early so that symptomatic treatment can be started, and any reversible causative factors identified and corrected.

The following case history illustrates the complexity of diagnosing and treating the confused patient.

Alex, a 45-year-old businessman who had previously enjoyed good health despite smoking 60 cigarettes a day, presented with headaches. Investigations showed lung cancer with multiple cerebral metastases. Treatment was immediately started with palliative radiotherapy to the brain, and dexamethasone 16 mg daily, given on an outpatient basis. A few days later, Alex's wife called his doctor out in the middle of the night. Having been increasingly restless and irritable since the diagnosis was made—and never having talked about it at home—he had refused to go to bed because he said he must urgently complete writing a computer programme 'to predict cosmic disintegration '. His wife found him swearing in frustration as he rapidly typed in a long list of commands which obviously made no sense. When she tried to calm him with a mug of hot chocolate, he threw it in her face. He had never behaved violently before.

(The change in Alex's mental state could result from biological factors: the cerebral tumours themselves, the side-effects of radiation or the side-effects of steroids. Psychological factors could be contributing too: it sounds as if he is avoiding, or

continued

continued

denying, open acknowledgement of his situation but symbolically expressing his sense of needing to complete his work before he dies. The psychodynamic concept of 'manic defence' could perhaps be relevant also.)

The doctor prescribed chlorpromazine 50 mg three times a day which seemed to make Alex worse; he became frankly confused, with slurred speech and incontinence of urine, continually climbing out of bed but then falling over, and striking out when people approached. He was admitted to hospital and his sedation changed to haloperidol, 10 mg at night and 5 mg twice daily, and his dexamethasone tapered down to 4 mg daily. A urinary infection was diagnosed, and antibiotics given for this.

Within a few days Alex became rational, and able to return home. When seen for followup he was no longer confused, and able to talk in a limited fashion about his situation. Though understandably despondent much of the time, he had been able to participate with some pleasure in various activities with his wife and family, and make plans with colleagues about the future of his firm. Two months later he died peacefully at home.

SOMATISATION

Somatisation can be defined as: 'a process in which there is inappropriate focus on physical symptoms, and psychosocial problems are denied '. There are obvious pitfalls in applying this concept with cancer patients, although it may well be quite common, and somatisation has not been well studied in oncology settings.

'Hypochondriasis', 'hysteria' and 'psychosomatic symptoms' are older terms with somewhat similar meaning.

Somatisation is frequent in the general population. Sometimes it is part of a psychiatric syndrome such as depression or anxiety. Other somatising patients do not have a formal psychiatric illness, but tend to respond to any stress in their lives by developing a physical symptom such as pain. Chronic somatisers may have gone the rounds of doctors, undergoing more and more elaborate medical investigations in a futile quest to discover an organic cause for their symptoms. Sometimes, although an organic basis has been found, the severity of the symptoms seems out of all proportion to it.

The tendency to somatise is influenced by cultural and family background, and by individual personality. Somatising patients often have difficulty acknowledging their feelings or finding the words to describe them. The physical symptom sometimes brings an advantage, such as care and attention from other people; and in many medical settings, somatisation is unwittingly encouraged by doctors and nurses who feel more comfortable with physical symptoms than emotional ones. A complaint about pain may well be treated more seriously and sympathetically than a complaint of feeling frightened or unhappy. True somatisation is not, however, the same thing as deliberate attention-seeking or malingering; somatising patients perceive their physical complaints as very real.

It is important that somatisation should be diagnosed on some positive psychological grounds, not merely invoked as a last resort when all the physical tests have drawn a blank.

In patients known to have a history of cancer, a diagnosis of somatisation must always be somewhat tentative, because there may well be a genuine and serious physical problem which has not yet shown up on examination or investigation. Many cancer patients claim they have been labelled 'neurotic' when their physical symptoms could not at first be explained, and have usually found this extremely hurtful, sometimes so much so that they refused to continue under the care of the doctor concerned. Such a breakdown of the therapeutic relationship could often have been avoided if the doctor had been more prepared to admit to uncertainty about the cause of the symptoms, and adopted more of a 'whole-person' approach to clinical problems.

When dealing with somatising patients, make it clear that their symptoms are regarded as genuine, while tactfully introducing the idea that psychological factors may be contributing. If basic physical investigations have been normal, it is best to call a halt to any further ones while a psychological approach is being pursued. Broaching the idea of referral to a psychiatrist or psychologist to some of these patients may seem a daunting task, yet must be presented honestly. Close collaboration between mental health professional and oncologist is essential, and a joint first consultation may be helpful.

Therapy will usually involve encouraging the patient to make links between emotional stresses and bodily symptoms. Many somatising patients have been brought up with the fixed belief that 'mental' and 'physical' matters are completely separate, and it may take persistence to educate them out of this view. Practical examples of making links include:

- Pointing out an obvious time relationship between unpleasant life events and the onset of physical symptoms, even if the patient was not aware of feeling upset about the events concerned.
- Pointing out the discrepancy between a patient's verbal denial of emotional distress, and non-verbal behaviour such as tearfulness.
- Explaining physiological mechanisms, such as the painful tensing of muscles which often accompanies anxiety.

While some patients will gladly accept permission to acknowledge their emotional distress, others will be hostile and defensive and may refuse to explore this aspect further. Psychological interpretations should not be forced upon the latter group; confrontation may alienate them for good, and it may be kinder to let them cling to their physical symptoms than exposing the underlying mental anguish.

FURTHER READING

Breitbart W. Suicide. In Holland JC, Rowland JH (eds) (1989) *Handbook of Psychooncology*. Oxford University Press: New York

Cody M (1990) Depression and the use of antidepressants in patients with cancer. *Palliative Medicine 4* 271–8

Faulkner A, Maguire P, Regnard C (1994). Dealing with anger in a patient or relative: a flow diagram. *Palliative Medicine 8* 51–57.

Fleishman SB, Lesko ML. Delirium and dementia. In Holland JC, Rowland JH (eds) (1989) *Handbook of Psychooncology*. Oxford University Press: New York

Greer S (1992). The management of denial in cancer patients. *Oncology 6* 33–40

Haig RA (1992) Management of depression in patients with advanced cancer. *Medical Journal of Australia 156* 499–503

Maguire P, Faulkner A, Regnard C (1993) Managing the anxious patient with advancing disease—a flow diagram. *Palliative Medicine 7* 239–44

Massie MJ. Anxiety, panic and phobias. In Holland JC, Rowland JH (eds) (1989) *Handbook of Psychooncology*. Oxford University Press: New York

Massie MJ Depression. In Holland JC, Rowland JH (eds) (1989) *Handbook of Psychooncology*. Oxford University Press: New York

Massie MJ, Holland JC. Overview of normal reactions and prevalence of psychiatric disorders. In Holland JC, Rowland JH (eds) (1989) *Handbook of Psychooncology*. Oxford University Press:New York

Mermelstein HT, Lesko LM (1992) Depression in patients with cancer *Psycho-oncology 1* 199–215

Saunders C (1992) Voluntary euthanasia. *Palliative Medicine 6* 1–5

Stedeford, A (1987) Confusion. In Bates T (ed) *Baillière's Clinical Oncology: Contemporary Palliation of Difficult Symptoms*. Baillière Tindall: London

Stedeford A, Regnard C (1991) Confusional states in advanced cancer—a flow diagram. *Palliative Medicine 5* 256–61

4
The Outcome of Cancer

At one end of the spectrum of possible longterm outcomes for patients with cancer is disease-free survival—at the other end is death.

For many patients, the outcome is not so clearly polarised. A few cancers have such an excellent prognosis that the word 'cure' may honestly be used following successful completion of treatment. More commonly, cure is a real possibility but cannot be guaranteed. Some patients whose cancer falls into this second category remain well for months or years following their primary treatment, but then develop a recurrence. This again may be treated successfully, or it may herald the development of widespread advanced disease. A further group of patients already have incurable cancer when first diagnosed, though such patients are not necessarily 'terminal' and may enjoy several more years of worthwhile life, depending on the type of cancer and whether it is responsive to treatment.

Although the physical features of a case will give some idea of prognosis, there is always some element of unpredictability and it is often impossible to say whether any given patient is going to survive the cancer or die from the disease. Nor can the timing of death be predicted accurately. Much interest has focused on whether psychological factors influence prognosis, and this complicated topic will be briefly considered here.

LONGTERM SURVIVAL (Tross and Holland 1989)

The experience of surviving cancer is perceived by some patients as a positive one which enhances their lives, by a few as a disastrous trauma which they never overcome, and by others as a temporary setback with little lasting impact.

Thanks to modern treatment techniques, many cancer patients now survive for years after diagnosis, and some can be considered permanently cured. The most striking improvements in prognosis have been achieved for certain lymphomas, leukaemias and solid tumours which develop in childhood and early adult life. However, the high doses of chemotherapy and/or radiotherapy necessary for the successful treatment of such conditions may result in permanent handicaps such as infertility or stunted growth.

The experience of having cancer at an early age might be expected to have a marked longterm psychological impact. Childhood cancer certainly has profound effects on whole families, but is outside the scope of this book. Regarding cancer in young adult life, several large followup surveys have been carried out on longterm survivors of Hodgkin's disease and testicular tumours, and show only small increases of psychiatric symptoms such as depression and anxiety, and social problems such as unemployment and divorce, over general population rates. Such surveys are reassuring in that they rule out gross psychosocial damage for the majority of patients. They may fail to detect the important but subtle changes in outlook—not necessarily undesirable ones—resulting from the cancer experience.

Positive psychological changes

Overall, at least 50% of patients successfully treated for cancer report some positive psychological changes. Enhanced appreciation of life; the art of living in the present; less concern for trivial or material things; more tolerance towards other people; improved self-confidence and self-worth are frequently reported. Such changes are illustrated by the following quotations, all from women who remained well two years following breast cancer surgery:

> 'I'm going to move house, change jobs and get things the way I want them—I mean to enjoy the rest of my life.'

> 'Now I can hold my own anywhere.'

> 'I've stopped worrying about housework or putting up a front.'

Negative Psychological Changes

A few patients remain haunted by fears of recurrent cancer even though they appear to have been cured. This is to some extent understandable, because cure can seldom be guaranteed.

These patients may adopt a permanent invalid role although they have no medical reason to do so, keep on constant watch for signs and symptoms of recurrence, and continue to brood over why they were singled out to develop cancer in the first place. TV programmes or magazine articles on cancer hold a morbid fascination for them. Routine outpatient appointments are reassuring for some, but for others serve to perpetuate their fears. One man wrote about his wife: 'She dreaded these clinic visits, which subjected her to tremendous strain for the two or three weeks leading up to what proved to be an hour's wait, a short examination and a perfunctory 'That's fine, see you again in six months.'' This reaction pattern, which has been called 'anxious preoccupation' or more colourfully the 'Damocles syndrome', may sometimes be helped by psychotherapy of the cognitive–behavioural variety, provided the patient recognises it as a problem and wants to change.

Social Stigma

Cancer survivors may encounter prejudice from acquaintances, neighbours, workmates, employers and insurance companies. While deliberate stigmatisation is rare, ignorance often causes needless damage. For example, many children and young adults miss out on education and employment following cancer treatment, because those in authority are misinformed—they assume such patients are bound to die in the near future, whereas in reality they may have an excellent prognosis.

Sometimes apparent prejudice exists largely in the patient's imagination. Many patients who have kept their diagnosis a secret at first, because they are afraid of being rejected, are pleasantly surprised by other people's warm acceptance if and when they do reveal the truth.

Late Side-effects of Treatment

Many of the side-effects of radiotherapy and chemotherapy clear up within a few weeks of completing the course of treatment, but if high doses have been used it may take several months for general well-being and energy to return to normal. Conditioned nausea and vomiting can prove especially persistent. New side-effects may develop some years after completion of high-dose radiotherapy and chemotherapy, usually due to fibrosis of the treated organs, and are occasionally highly disabling both physically and emotionally.

Annabel, the 35-year-old manageress of a fashion boutique, received radical radiotherapy for treatment of cervical cancer. Treatment was successful in the sense of eradicating the tumour but fibrosis of the pelvic organs, due to unusually severe radiation side-effects, caused recurrent complications over the next few years, culminating in the need for a colostomy. This procedure was repugnant to Annabel, who felt her 'body image' and sense of femininity had been irretrievably destroyed. Her former 'fighting spirit' attitude was replaced by a 'helpless–hopeless' one, she virtually stopped eating and drinking, and openly stated that she wished to die. Psychotherapy and antidepressants made no impact. Weakened by weight loss and prolonged bed rest, she developed a fatal chest infection.

Such tragic cases are very rare. Much more often, late side-effects seem a small price to pay for curing the cancer. This is not to imply that patients should quietly put up with their symptoms for fear of appearing ungrateful—it is important that late side-effects should be brought to medical attention. There may be simple ways to help patients already affected, for example the use of massage, skin care and bandaging for the limb swelling (lymphoedema) which may follow surgery and/or radiotherapy, or lubricants and dilators for radiation-induced narrowing of the vagina. And for those other patients yet to be treated in the future, there may be ways to prevent late side-effects developing at all. With the current emphasis on 'quality of life', it is recognised that new treatment techniques should seek to minimise side-effects—both early and late—as well as achieving better rates of cancer cure.

ADVANCED CANCER: PALLIATIVE CARE (Cassidy 1986; Stedeford 1994; Twycross 1992)

Some of the topics discussed in detail elsewhere in this book are reconsidered here in relation to patients whose illness has reached its terminal stage, and whose life expectancy is only a few weeks or months.

Emotional Adjustment to Advanced Cancer

Advanced cancer may demand great emotional adjustment, because of the unpleasant physical symptoms and the lack of any realistic prospect of recovery. The classic sequence of denial, anger, despair and acceptance may be repeated over again when a patient learns that the cancer has become incurable. Some patients who have already achieved an attitude of acceptance when first diagnosed can maintain this. Others, who have previously acknowledged what is wrong with them, lapse back into denial to cope with this extra stress.

Patients with stable personalities, a satisfying past life and strong support from their families and friends generally adjust more readily to terminal illness than those whose former existence was of a troubled kind. Exceptions are found. Facing death may be especially difficult for those who have a great deal to lose by dying, such as young people who have not yet achieved their full potential, or those utterly unaccustomed to the 'sick role'. For example, a formerly active and successful businessman who is used to being in charge at work, and filling his leisure time with active sports, has a tremendous adjustment to make in the face of terminal cancer.

Emotional Problems of Terminal Illness

Adjusting to loss: the multiple losses already discussed in relation to a cancer diagnosis are seen in particularly stark form. Further losses may be added: elderly patients no longer able to cope alone may have to leave their homes or give up much-loved pets, and younger patients be forced to retire from work. *Physical weakness* often becomes so marked as to deprive the patient of activities and independence. Some find this humiliating, and are greatly concerned about burdening others. The enforced *loss of role* can lead to boredom, and sometimes causes friction with those who have had to take over the patient's former duties. *Body image* changes often include altered size or shape, and sometimes visible tumour on exposed parts. Loss of *ability to communicate*, for those patients who are dysphasic or dysarthric because of lesions in the brain or larynx, is frustrating and distressing especially for those who clearly know what they want to say but cannot make themselves understood. Loss of future *life expectancy* and of *control over future destiny* can give rise to much distress.

Communication about the illness with relatives and staff may be difficult. Telling children is especially hard. These problems add to the sense of *alienation* from healthy people which many dying patients experience. Some gradually withdraw from those around them. This can be upsetting to relatives who, not realising it is a natural prelude to death, feel personally rejected.

Depression is a significant problem for about one-quarter of patients admitted for hospice care. Clinical depression is difficult to distinguish from the symptoms of the cancer itself, from the appropriate sadness associated with dying, and from the 'weariness of life' which may contribute to lethargy and withdrawal in patients whose illness has dragged on a long time. Useful pointers to clinical depression include: prominent feelings of being a burden to others, inability to enjoy things which *could* still bring pleasure (a favourite TV programme, visits from relatives), thoughts of suicide or euthanasia, and pain which does not respond to the usual measures. (Poorly controlled pain is itself a potent source of depression.) Antidepressant drugs help in some cases, and their hypnotic and analgesic properties may be a useful bonus. However, they may cause unwanted effects such as sedation, dry mouth, and constipation. There is no need to rush into the prescription of antidepressants for patients admitted to a hospice, because mood sometimes lifts rapidly in response to the caring environment.

Anxiety is also found in about a quarter of patients, often combined with depression. At root, it is probably related to the fear of death, though not all patients can acknowledge or articulate this fear—instead, they may pin their anxiety on trivial things, or express it by frequent demands for nursing attention. Anxiety is often worse at night, or when the patient is alone. Some are afraid to go to sleep, perhaps because they fear they will never wake up; others are troubled by nightmares. If the patient can recognise the source of the fears, and talk about this, it usually helps. There may be a specific worry which is largely unfounded, for example about bleeding or choking to death in cases where this is unlikely.

Confusion, often due to a combination of metabolic disturbance and medication, is common in the last few weeks of life. *Terminal agitation*, in which features of delirium are combined with those of acute anxiety, is occasionally found in patients who have not managed to come to terms with the diagnosis of incurable illness or with other problems from their past.

Freda, a 65-year-old widow of anxious personality, had had haematuria for many months before she consulted her doctor. Investigation showed an advanced carcinoma of the bladder. She came into the hospice because of attacks of trembling and tightness in the chest, on account of which she had been phoning her doctor's surgery several times each day. No physical cause for her symptoms was found and Freda herself thought they were due to being alone. The attacks diminished after a few days, and discharge home was discussed, but she then developed nausea

continued

continued

and chest pain for which no organic cause was apparent. Then, Freda suddenly became acutely disturbed. She had never talked to the staff about her illness or asked about her prognosis, but one day she suddenly yelled out 'I've got cancer and I'm going to die!' and began to weep inconsolably. When staff tried to comfort her she pushed them away, demanding to be taken into hospital and apparently not believing she was already there. Misperceptions were evident, for example she pointed at her jacket and said another woman was in the room. She begged to see her son, from whom she had been estranged for many years. With difficulty the ward staff managed to trace him, and with even more difficulty persuaded him to visit his dying mother, but Freda did not recognise him when he came.

Religious and spiritual issues: formalised religion, and/or belief in an afterlife, is a major source of comfort to some patients but not to all. A few believers lose their faith at this time, whereas a few agnostics undergo a religious conversion. 'Spiritual' issues are broader than religious ones and include a quest for meaning in the illness; resolution of old conflicts; and integration of past life experience.

Management

Palliative surgery, chemotherapy and especially *radiotherapy* may achieve worthwhile relief of symptoms in terminal patients, and sometimes an extension of lifespan, but these gains must be balanced against the side-effects, inconvenience and cost of treatment. A time will come when it is best to discontinue specific anticancer treatment and concentrate on relieving symptoms like pain, sleeplessness or anxiety. Deciding when this time has arrived is not always easy.

Determination to continue treatment right to the end may be a positive decision which reflects a 'fighting spirit' and merits respect. For other patients, stopping treatment would be too painful an acknowledgement that the disease is beyond cure.

Doctors as well as patients can think this way. Other patients want to continue because of an extreme fear of death, or a sense of guilt about 'giving up' and letting the family down.

The decision to stop treatment may be perfectly reasonable in the case of patients who realise that death is inevitable and prefer to spend the rest of their lives quietly with the minimum of medical intervention. Other patients want to give up prematurely because for some reason they welcome the prospect of death, perhaps as a means of escape from unhappy personal circumstances. It is always worth exploring the individual's motives in the case of an apparently misguided decision, as certain problems may be remediable ones.

Control of physical symptoms is closely linked to the management of emotional distress in the terminally ill. Emotional issues in dying patients can only be satisfactorily addressed when the physical symptoms are reasonably well controlled. Paradoxically, however, successful relief of physical suffering may have the effect of unmasking emotional distress of which the patient was previously unaware. And when physical symptoms prove unusually difficult to control, it may be that they represent a substitute for emotional distress ('*somatisation*'), as illustrated by the case of Freda above.

The drugs commonly used for symptom control include a number of psychotropic agents. Haloperidol helps both vomiting and anxiety; amitriptyline helps depression, insomnia and pain. Terminal cancer patients are often on many different drugs, so there is a risk of drug interactions, or mistakes in dosage.

Practical aids, ranging from the simple (a wig; some large-print books) to the sophisticated (an electric wheelchair), can restore morale and mobility and so improve mood.

Counselling and psychotherapy must be short-term, and not unduly ambitious in their aims, although some patients are able to achieve marked psychological change in a short period of time. It is difficult to keep to a pure theoretical model or a rigid treatment schedule. The therapist must be flexible enough to change appointment times, or vary the length of sessions, to fit in with medical treatments or with day-to-day changes in the patient's state. A patient who is drowsy and mildly confused on one day may be eager to participate in a detailed discussion the next. Human warmth is of more value than intellectual sophistication and sometimes it seems right to breach the conventions of therapy, for example by holding a patient's hand.

The Hospice Movement

Until about twenty years ago there was scant provision for patients suffering from advanced cancer or other forms of terminal illness. Now palliative care has become a recognised medical specialty. Alternative terms include terminal care, continuing care and hospice care. Most patients treated in palliative care units have cancer, but similar principles apply to certain other chronic illnesses such as neurological conditions and AIDS.

Dame Cicely Saunders, founder and first medical director of St Christopher's Hospice, London, has done much to develop work in this field. Hospices, including both National Health Service (NHS) units and independent foundations supported by charitable funds, have pioneered improvements in the care of dying patients and, through teaching programmes, raised the profile of palliative care work.

Control of physical symptoms such as pain, nausea and breathlessness is an important part of palliative care but in parallel with this, high priority is given to the psychological, social and spiritual issues affecting patients, relatives and staff. The aims of treatment do not include cure, nor necessarily the prolongation of life. More important goals are the relief of distressing symptoms, and helping both patient and family to make the most of the life which remains. Care is continued as long as it is needed, which is usually until the death of the patient and often longer, if the family need ongoing support.

Hospices are not merely places to die. Many patients are admitted for a week or so to achieve improved control of symptoms, or to give their families a rest, and then return home. Most hospices have facilities for day patient care; specialist community nursing sisters (Macmillan nurses) who visit patients and their families at home and liaise with their primary care teams; and a bereavement service to provide followup support to relatives. Volunteers as well as professionals contribute to patient care, and there is emphasis on multidisciplinary team work.

The following history illustrates the team management of a complicated case.

Jacqueline, 38, had advanced ovarian cancer. Following an unsuccessful course of chemotherapy she was admitted to the hospice, nauseated and weak. She was unwilling to give any medical history, saying resentfully 'I just don't feel well that's all' and 'I've been through it all so many times before.'

The sympathy felt by the staff towards this young woman became strained to its limits over the following week as Jacqueline seemed to reject all their best efforts. She said 'This isn't like a proper medical ward where they do treatments—I came here to recuperate but this place is just making me worse.' She complained that her room was too noisy and too hot, but when given a different one, complained of the cold and isolation. She criticised the food and asked for prawn sandwiches, but when a nurse prepared these she left them untouched, saying she might have fancied something hot. When her gynaecology consultant postponed his planned visit for a day, because of emergency surgery on another patient, she said 'Everyone lets me down—I'm being pushed around from pillar to post.'

Jacqueline's nausea was brought under control with drugs. She was found to be anaemic and received a blood transfusion. With some reluctance, she agreed to daily exercises supervised by the physiotherapist, and to relaxation training with the occupational therapist.

As the psychiatrist attached to the ward, I was also asked to see Jacqueline. I found her unreceptive at first, resentful towards me and unwilling to talk, but visited her daily for short periods in the hope of building up some rapport. I also spent some time discussing her case with other staff, some of whom had started to describe her as 'difficult' or 'manipulative', not realising that the awkward behaviour represented a projection of fear and anger about the advancing disease. When I felt Jacqueline herself had developed a little confidence in me, I suggested some of this to her directly; she admitted how insecure she felt with the changes of ward and changes of staff, and how bitterly envious of the cheerful healthy young nurses.

continued

continued

Soon after she started to talk more openly in this way, Jacqueline became frankly depressed; lying in bed with no interest in anything, but complaining of inner feelings of panic and tension. After she had been in this state for a few days I prescribed her an antidepressant drug (paroxetine 20 mg daily). During the week which followed she talked much more freely; telling of her past life as a happy active person who loved her job with an airline, but of her recent 'bad luck' when both her parents had died, her flat had been burgled and her boyfriend left, all about the same time as the cancer developed. She wept when reviewing all these losses. From being an aggressively independent patient when she arrived on the ward, she became rather the opposite, showing an almost child-like gratitude for whatever the staff did for her.

About ten days after starting the antidepressant, a very clear improvement was evident in Jacqueline's mood. At the same time she put renewed efforts into her walking, with some success, and her general condition improved so much that she was able to spend a day visiting a friend's home and greatly enjoyed it.

Another week, however, brought a rapid decline in her physical condition. She asked for some blood tests and X-rays to be repeated 'so I know where I am and can make proper arrangements'. The results confirmed the clinical deterioration and, aware 'my days are numbered', she asked the ward social worker to arrange for a solicitor to visit. Jacqueline wrote her will, and asked her friends to come and see her for the last time. She died peacefully a few days later.

DO PSYCHOLOGICAL FACTORS AFFECT CANCER GROWTH? (Holland 1989)

The prime causes of cancer are biological. Many factors including genetic make-up, diet, smoking, virus infection and exposure to radiation or certain chemicals are known to influence the onset and course of the disease. However, such factors only provide a partial explanation. Given the present state of knowledge it is not possible to say why, for example, one heavy smoker develops lung cancer while another escapes; or why one woman treated for breast cancer makes a full recovery while another, whose case is apparently similar, develops distant metastases and dies within a few months. Many people believe that psychological factors like attitude to illness, or experience of stress, could be involved. This is a complicated topic, also a controversial one which often arouses strong feelings and opposing views.

Some research studies on this subject are based on interviews designed to explore the personality, mood and life histories of cancer patients as compared with healthy people. Others involve laboratory measurements of biological variables, such as immune function and hormone secretion, which could mediate links between cancer and the mind; some of this work has been carried out on animals subjected to stressful conditions. The term 'psychoneuroimmunology' describes this field of research.

Conflicting findings have emerged from the work so far completed. Those studies yielding 'positive' results have excited most interest, but review of the published literature reveals many carefully-done, but less well-known, studies with negative findings. Providing a thorough review of present knowledge would require a detailed discussion of research methods and of individual papers, beyond the scope of this book. The brief summary presented here can do little more than indicate the complexity of the subject!

The Variables of Interest

Personality: perhaps the most consistent findings relate to the personality traits of patients with cancer. The key characteristic, as identified by several independent research groups, is the denial and/or repression of emotions such as anger, resentment, hostility or aggressiveness. This profile has been called the 'Type C personality'. Type C people come over as unusually 'nice' and anxious to please, put others' needs before their own, and are reluctant to complain. The simplistic interpretation, that a lifetime of bottling up real feelings has caused the development of cancer, can only be speculation. It must also be emphasised that this description does not by any means apply to all patients with cancer, and that overall differences on personality scales for cancer patients compared with healthy people are small ones.

Mood: the findings here are less clearcut. Some studies have reported a raised rate of cancer in people with high scores on depression scales completed many years earlier; other studies have failed to confirm these findings. 'Prodromal' depression has been described as an early manifestation of cancer, especially pancreatic cancer. It is not clear whether this represents anything more than a chance association between two common conditions; or, if a true association does exist, whether the cancer or the depression came first. One theory would be that immune deficiency associated with depression permits a latent cancer to grow more quickly; another, that occult cancer produces depressive symptoms through some neurochemical disturbance. Depressive symptoms are, however, difficult to distinguish from those of cancer itself. Somewhat at variance with these reports are several studies on the prognosis of established cancer, showing that patients who become depressed following their diagnosis tend to live longer than others.

Life event stress: the longstanding belief that adverse life events, especially those involving the loss of a close relationship, are conducive to cancer has attracted renewed interest in recent years with the discovery that immune function becomes impaired following bereavement. In theory, this could increase susceptibility to cancer. However, there is very little clinical evidence that bereaved people actually do have a raised cancer risk. Large case-record studies have, for example, demonstrated exactly the same lifetime frequency of widowhood and divorce in breast cancer patients as in healthy women. Interview studies, which can also take other types of life event into account, have given conflicting results. Patients in whom the onset or recurrence of cancer follows soon after an adverse life event are clinically striking, but adverse life events are very common, and such cases may represent mere coincidence.

Social support: a strong network of personal relationships might be expected to protect against developing cancer, or improve the prognosis of cancer. Some research studies, but not others, provide evidence for this effect.

Attitude to disease: several studies have reported that the best prognosis is found in patients with a 'fighting spirit' attitude, and the worst prognosis in those with a 'helpless–hopeless' one.

All these variables are to some degree interlinked, but most studies have only attempted to examine one at once, otherwise the exercise would become impossibly cumbersome.

How Might a Link be Explained?

Showing the existence of a link between some psychological factor and cancer does not necessarily mean a cause-and-effect relationship, though many people assume that this is so. Possible explanations include:

- Direct biological cause-and-effect through mechanisms which would presumably involve immunological or hormonal change.
- Indirect cause-and-effect through changes in behaviour. Behaviours such as smoking, drinking, sunbathing and sexual promiscuity, all of which are linked to certain forms of cancer, depend both on individual psychology and on social circumstances. So do compliance with healthcare advice and medical treatment.
- The psychological change could be caused by the cancer rather than the other way round, for example the helpless–hopeless attitude may indicate that a heavy tumour burden is already present even if not clinically detectable.
- Chance coexistence: adverse life events, and episodes of depression, are common within the general population and are sometimes bound to coincide in time with the onset of cancer.
- Genetic linkage: certain personality characteristics, or a vulnerability to depression, might go together with vulnerability to cancer.
- An apparent link might be invalid, due to the methodological problems listed below.

Problems of Investigating the Field

These include:

- Assessing psychological variables: instruments to measure personality, mood, or experience of stress are not 100% valid or reliable even in physically healthy people, and may be considerably less satisfactory for patients suffering from cancer.

- Memory bias and 'effort after meaning': patients' memories are often inaccurate especially if they already know or suspect their diagnosis and are striving to find an explanantion for becoming ill.
- Timing: because there is no way of timing the onset of a cancer in clinical practice, whether the cancer began before or after a given psychological stressor cannot be known.
- Choice of a comparison / control group: hospital patients with non-cancerous conditions are not typical of the general population, yet for example women with benign breast lumps are often used for comparison purposes in psychological studies of breast cancer.

All these problems are particularly marked with retrospective studies—that is, studies in which interviews take place after the cancer has already developed. Prospective studies are more time-consuming and complicated to carry out, because they require a large number of healthy people to be followed up for many years until some of them develop cancer, and few sound prospective studies on this topic have been done.

Clinical Implications

The concept of a link between emotional factors and cancer growth is attractive to many people. It seems to provide an intuitively appealing explanation for a mysterious disease, and offer scope for patients to influence the future outcome by taking control of their lifestyle and emotions.

Links between behavioural factors, such as smoking, and development of cancer are well-established and clinically important. As regards more direct causative links between psychological variables and cancer, the truth is far from clear. Even if the existence of such links was proven—which at present is not the case—it does not follow that trying to alter psychological factors is a feasible prospect, or that doing so would make any difference to cancer risk or outcome.

Personality characteristics, by definition, are an integral part of psychological make-up and can seldom be changed very much. Stressful life events—bereavement for example—inevitably form part of most people's experience and their adverse impact can only be partly softened by the most skilled counselling and the best social support.

Clumsy over-simplifications of the kind of theories outlined above are often bandied about in the popular media and, far from benefiting patients, can magnify suffering for themselves and their families. Thinking 'I've got a cancer-prone personality' or 'This illness came on because my husband left me' or 'It's my own fault I'm getting worse—I'm not being positive enough' is likely to make patients feel guilty or bitter and is no help to them at all. There is a danger that patients who think this way will invest too high hopes, and sometimes too much time and money, in trying to change—only to blame themselves if their cancer progresses all the same.

The statements above are not intended to devalue the other benefits of psychological interventions for cancer patients. Cultivation of a positive attitude, learning relaxation and stress management techniques, any of the whole range of complementary therapies designed to enhance physical and mental wellbeing, are desirable if they help patients feel better, or adjust more easily to their illness. Whether such therapies can make any difference to the actual outcome of the cancer, however, is a separate question to which the answer is unknown.

Summary and Comment

Despite much research effort, the role of psychological factors in cancer growth remains unclear. If they had a major effect it would probably have become plain by now. Although the evidence is so conflicting, many people are convinced that psychological factors do play a role in the course of cancer and that good emotional support, learning to cope with stress and adopting a 'fighting-spirit' attitude are essential for survival. This approach is helpful in some cases but counter-productive in others. Lifestyle and attitude changes should be encouraged if they help patients cope better with their cancer diagnosis—but not presented as a cure for the cancer itself.

FURTHER READING

Cassidy S (1986) Emotional distress in terminal cancer: discussion paper. *Journal of the Royal Society of Medicine 79* 717–20

Holland JC. Behavioural and psychosocial risk factors in cancer: human studies. In Holland JC, Rowland JH (eds) (1989) *Handbook of Psychooncology*. Oxford University Press: New York

Stedeford A (1984) *Facing Death*. Oxford: Heinemann (1994 edition in press: Sobell Publications. Available from Sir Michael Sobell House, Churchill Hospital, Oxford OX3 7LJ)

Tross S, Holland JC. Psychological sequelae in cancer survivors. In Holland JC, Rowland JH (eds) (1989) *Handbook of Psychooncology*. Oxford University Press: New York

Twycross RG (1992) Editorial: care of the terminally ill patient. *Triangle 31* 1–7

5
Emotional Issues for Families

This part of the book is about the cancer patient's relatives and friends—who may be just as much emotionally affected by the illness as the patient, sometimes more. Provision for family needs should form part of any good cancer treatment service. Nurses and social workers, whether based in the hospital or in primary care, and general practitioners are key contributors to this service.

The patient's partner—spouse or cohabitee—is usually the main carer in both emotional and practical terms. Sometimes this role is taken by a parent, child, sibling or friend instead. A few patients have no close relatives or friends and may depend entirely on healthcare professionals, and on their fellow-patients, for support.

Problems which may arise between couples—communication barriers, sexual dysfunction, role changes, mood disorder in the partner—will be considered here, also the problems which face the children of parents with cancer. Bereavement is also considered in this section.

Occasional families have all these problems and more. When unhapppy relationships, social deprivation, and poor mental and physical health have already been present for years, the advent of cancer in one family member may precipitate complete chaos. Professional helpers may feel overwhelmed unless they recognise the boundaries of their own roles, and set realistic limits on what they can hope to achieve.

While cancer in one family member almost inevitably does create problems of some kind for the others, it is also common to see couples and families brought closer together by the cancer experience. Patient and carer often come to appreciate one another more deeply, learn to talk about issues which were too difficult before, and find unsuspected personal strengths in dealing with the illness (Rait and Lederberg 1989; Smith and Regnard 1993).

CHANGES FOR COUPLES

Communication Barriers

Paradoxically, communication problems can be most troublesome in happy families, for whom talking about cancer and the possibility of dying is most likely to cause pain. Well-meaning attempts to protect one's partner from the diagnosis altogether can lead to a complex web of concealment. There is an apocryphal story of a cancer patient and his wife who came together to the outpatient clinic, each asking to see the doctor alone. The husband said 'I know it's cancer but you mustn't tell my wife.' The wife said 'I know it's cancer but you mustn't tell my husband.' What the doctor did is not recorded.

Another (real) case had a satisfactory outcome.

Jack, a rather inarticulate man in his early 60s, had small cell lung cancer. The diagnosis was initially given to his wife, who insisted he must not be told. Every time Jack came to hospital for chemo-therapy she came too, and asked to see the doctor first, to remind him not to mention the diagnosis. One day she was not able to do this and the doctor, assuming Jack already knew what was wrong, casually mentioned the word 'cancer' to him. When she found out what had happened, Jack's wife created an emotional scene but after that, the couple were able to talk to each other much more easily. Jack said he was very pleased to know and his wife admitted it was a big relief.

Cases like this still occur, even though most doctors nowadays favour disclosing a cancer diagnosis to the patient directly, and relatives have no official right to veto this.

Even when both partners know the diagnosis, they may not discuss it very much with one another. Some couples do not need to; having acknowledged the situation to begin with, and dealt with any necessary practicalities, the understanding is in place and they may be providing strong support for one another without the need for words. This way of coping should not be disturbed if both partners are content with it.

Less satisfactory are those situations in which the communication needs of the two partners are different. One woman with advanced lung cancer said in exasperation 'I've tried to make my husband realise what I've got but he won't listen. The one time I did get through, he broke right down. I don't know how he's going to cope when I've gone.' Far from supporting one another, such couples are adding to each other's distress. Sometimes they can be helped by joint interviews with a skilled person to understand each other's views and needs, and share some of their emotions.

Sexual Problems (Auchincloss 1989)

Sexual problems among patients with cancer are often ignored, partly because of the general reticence which surrounds sexual topics in our society and partly because of an assumption that sex is a minor issue for those with such a serious physical disease.

Many doctors and nurses never even consider the sexual aspect of their patients' lives, and others are too embarrassed to broach the subject. However, it is an increasingly important one, now that more young patients with cancer can expect to survive for long periods. Several factors contribute to sexual problems:

- *Physical changes* due to surgical or radiation damage, hormone therapy or cytotoxic drugs, can lead to impotence and/or infertility. Partial recovery sometimes takes place over a period of several months.
- *Body image changes*, both general ones such as weight change or hair loss and those with a more direct bearing on sexuality (mastectomy, orchidectomy, procedures on the bladder or bowel), often inhibit sexual activity for psychological reasons. The patient feels unattractive, even physically repellent.

Sometimes of course the partner feels the same way—one man, accompanying his wife to the outpatient consultation at which the recommendation for mastectomy was made, told the surgeon 'A woman with one breast will be no —ing use to me.' This attitude is fortunately unusual. Most partners would be willing and able to adapt to the patient's changed body if given the chance.

- *Relationship changes* between the couple concerned can inhibit sexuality. One typical sequence of events is that the healthy partner refrains from making any sexual overtures, out of concern for the sick person, who takes this as a rejection and feels even more unattractive. Neither partner likes to make the first move. In another common pattern the change from an equal relationship between two healthy adults, to a carer/patient relationship more akin to that between parent and child, does not seem conducive to sex.
- *Mistaken beliefs*, for example that cancer can be transmitted to a sexual partner, or that intercourse and/or pregnancy will damage the patient, may inhibit sexual activity. In some cases such beliefs contain at least a core of truth, in others they are inaccurate.

Patients living in a happy and stable partnership may be able to adapt to impairments of sexual function. Though full intercourse declines, other kinds of physical contact in the form of kisses or cuddles may increase, and the general relationship between the couple grow closer. Other patients, however, suffer much unhappiness because of the effect of cancer on their sexual functioning. The overall quality of a marriage, not just its sexual aspect, may deteriorate. Patients without a current partner may feel unable to embark on new relationships.

Management must start with disclosure of the problem and, because so many patients are reticent about sexual topics, the doctor or nurse needs to ask direct questions. Seeing both partners together is a good idea, and may enable them to talk openly about the problem for the first time. Misunderstandings can be corrected and accurate factual information given. The couple may be advised to set aside regular time, daily or every few days, to be together in private and exchange affection through words and touch, but making no attempt to have intercourse. For couples who have drifted apart emotionally, this apparently simple exercise will help to re-establish mutual trust and communication.

Fertility and contraception are related topics, also frequently neglected. Fertility in patients undergoing treatment for cancer is likely to be reduced but not always abolished. Pregnancy would usually be unwelcome at this time, because of uncertainty about prognosis of the cancer and/or fears that chemotherapy or radiotherapy could damage the unborn child. Staff should take the initiative in discussing contraception with patients of childbearing age. Later on, however, if treatment for the cancer has been completed successfully, many young patients will be hopeful of starting a family. They may be encouraged to learn that there is no excess risk of congenital abnormalities in babies born to young adult survivors of anticancer treatment. Less happily, the fertility of many such survivors is low. For young male patients, anticipation of this issue may permit sperm banking to be carried out before chemotherapy or radiotherapy begins. Another consideration is that some types of cancer are inherited; genetic counselling, individualised for particular families, permits an estimate of the risk of any children being affected in the future. For patients who are physically unable to conceive normally, or who decide against trying because the risks are too high, various techniques of assisted conception might be considered although these are not widely available under the NHS.

Information about likely changes in sexuality and reproductive function can be included in leaflets prepared for patients about to undergo standardised treatments for cancer.

Heightened sex drive in cancer patients is an infrequent problem but sometimes highly distressing. It may arise in men or women given androgenic drugs, or be a manifestation of disinhibited behaviour in patients with organic brain disease, perhaps representing a form of over-compensation for the loss of sexual powers.

In summary, issues of sexuality should always be addressed for younger patients, if only because of the contraceptive aspect, and closer attention to this topic would often be welcome for older patients too.

Role Changes

Role changes are enforced when the person with cancer is physically limited, whether temporarily by intensive treatment for early cancer, or permanently by advancing disease. Within the traditional family, a sick husband becomes unable to go to work, drive the car, do household repairs or tend the garden; whereas a sick wife can no longer manage housework, cooking, shopping and child care. At the same time as coping with great emotional stress, the healthy partner has to take over unfamiliar practical responsibilities. There may well be extra demands, such as relatives coming to stay, or long journeys to and from hospital; and fewer resources to meet these demands, for example interrupted sleep night after night, and less money coming in because one or both partners have been forced to stop work.

Most carers are very willing to look after their sick loved one, and feel rewarded by an improved sense of purpose and a closer intimacy. But the role of carer inevitably carries some strain.

Flexibility is a great asset in coping with the enforced changes. Some couples, even elderly ones whose traditional roles have been sharply demarcated throughout their married life, see the situation as an opportunity or challenge. The wife learns to drive, or the husband learns to cook, and both partners take pride in the new skill. Others feel threatened by the prospect of change. The sick partner deeply resents the loss of role, and is convinced that nobody else can take over to a proper standard. A common example is the husband who, no longer able to drive the car himself, resorts to constant criticism of his wife's driving style.

It is important in trying to avoid this type of response that patients do not feel deprived of any useful role at all, even if they can no longer fulfil their previous one. The man confined to a wheelchair can no longer do heavy physical work, but could perhaps take over responsibility for the household accounts.

A few patients complain that their partners make little or no allowance for their illness, and expect them to carry on as before. Sometimes this does reflect a thoughtless selfishness in the partner, or it may be evidence of denial—the partner would find it so painful to acknowledge the patient's condition that he or she plays it down, unwittingly coming over as inconsiderate or callous.

Carers face the difficult challenge of striking the right balance, neither expecting too much from patients nor wrapping them in cotton wool, always bearing in mind that patients' capabilities can vary during the course of an illness, and even dying patients can have 'good days'.

Eliza, a 55-year-old housewife recently diagnosed with advanced breast cancer, was upset and angry when her family failed to visit her in hospital one weekend. Her distress deepened when she learned the reason: they had been decorating her bedroom. They had meant this as a surprise treat, but her reaction was to feel left out, and deprived of her role in the household. She seemed determined to dislike whatever wallpaper they had chosen. Following several meetings with the patient, family and ward staff, Eliza and her relatives acknowledged their need to talk directly to each other about the shock of the diagnosis and the changes that her illness would mean in their daily lives. Before Eliza went home she remarked 'I can see now they all meant well—and I'm still just as important to them, but in a different way. We've all got to learn to go with the tide."

Mood Disorders in Carers

Research surveys show that depression and anxiety are almost as common among patients' partners as among patients themselves. This means that about half the partners will have some symptoms, and in up to a quarter these will be severe. There tends to be concordance between patient and partner; that is, if one is emotionally distressed, the other is likely to be so too. However, this distress has often not been shared because each partner is trying so hard not to upset the other.

The partner's emotional response may be complicated by anger or guilt, often indicating some past conflict in the relationship. Sometimes cancer acts as the catalyst for resolution of longstanding marital problems, but sometimes a shaky marriage breaks down completely under the extra strain.

If emotional problems in patients themselves are frequently not recognised, this is even more likely to be so for those in their carers, who often feel obliged to keep cheerful and put on a brave face. It is helpful if carers can be seen alone from time to time, perhaps by the family doctor, asked how they are coping and invited to talk over any emotional distress. It is also sometimes helpful if this can be followed by a joint interview including the patient, to encourage sharing of mutual grief and distress.

Carers most severely affected may benefit from formal counselling and/or a course of psychotropic drugs.

Practical Help for Carers

In the case of an incurable cancer patient being looked after at home, the burden on the carer may be heavy and prolonged. All carers deserve a break occasionally, and may need permission and encouragement to go out alone or with friends and enjoy a favourite activity, even something of an apparently frivolous kind like having a hairdo or playing sport. However devoted and competent the carer may be, he (or more often she) cannot be expected to cope singlehanded all the time. Professional services should never be completely withheld because there is an able-bodied carer in the household; this is an exploitation of the carer. Home visits by such professionals as district nurses, Macmillan nurses, Marie Curie nurses, occupational therapists, physiotherapists, social workers, care assistants and others should ensure that all available help is being provided. Regular respite care in hospital for the patient, preferably on a regular basis (say one week in every six), and regular visits to a day centre, may be invaluable in sustaining the carer through a long period of hard physical work and mental distress.

CHILDREN OF CANCER PATIENTS (Couldrick 1988, 1991)

Although the majority of cancer patients are middle-aged or elderly, others are young enough to have children still at home. Telling children about the illness is often a difficult and painful task.

Telling is hardest of all in cases with a poor prognosis, when the affected parent is likely to become gradually worse and eventually die. In such cases, however, it is almost always desirable for children to be given some explanation of what is already happening, and some preparation for what is to come.

Children below the age of about seven may not be capable of understanding the finality of death, especially if this is something to be anticipated in the future rather than a completed event. Understanding is easier for those who have seen the topic portrayed on TV, or personally experienced the loss of a grandparent or a pet. Some young children indeed show a surprisingly matter-of-fact interest and acceptance; wanting to dig up the body of a buried dog or cat is a common example.

With teenagers, despite their fuller intellectual understanding, communication on this sensitive subject may be even more difficult than it is with younger children, because adolescence is so often a time of emotional turmoil when parents and children find it hard to talk to each other anyway.

As a general rule, children of all ages tend to know and understand more than their parents give them credit for, or perhaps want to believe. Trying to keep children in complete ignorance of a parent's illness is most unlikely to work, although it may make the parents themselves feel more comfortable. Even when the subject is never talked about at home, a child's distress will often be plain through physical symptoms or changes in behaviour, for example:

- Becoming 'clingy' and crying over small upsets.
- Poor appetite, abdominal pain, vomiting.
- Sleep disturbance and bad dreams.
- Wetting or soiling.
- Exacerbation of asthma, skin rashes, headaches.
- Refusing to go to school, or low achievement at school.
- Aggressive or destructive behaviour.

Besides the obvious emotion of grief, children may feel angry about being abandoned by the sick parent, irrationally guilty about somehow being responsible for the illness, or frightened that cancer will develop in their other parent or in themselves. Some children feel obliged to take over the role of a sick parent of the same sex. Encouraging a boy to become 'the man of the family', or a girl 'a mother to the little ones' can place a heavy burden on a grieving child, though many children assume this burden of their own accord and take on responsibilities beyond their years.

How a child reacts depends a great deal on surrounding circumstances; how much support is given by the healthy parent and other relatives and friends, and whether the sick parent's illness has caused practical deprivations such as shortage of money or an enforced move of house. Consistent care from a trusted adult, even if not a biological relative, is very important. Consistent domestic routine, with regular mealtimes and bedtimes, can help provide a sense of security. The child should be allowed, even encouraged, to talk about the parent's illness, and ask questions to which honest answers are given.

It can sometimes be easier for somebody outside the family to talk to a child. Some specialised nurses, including Macmillan nurses, have expertise in this field, as do some general practitioners, social workers, counsellors in medical settings, and priests. Teachers can often help and it is certainly a good idea for them to know about the situation, which is bound to have some effect on the child's school work and relationship with classmates. Booklets and videos exist to help children's understanding, though it is difficult for any single version to cater adequately for all age-groups.

Children should not be excluded if and when the parent's condition gets worse. They should be encouraged to visit in hospital and, should the parent die, have the opportunity to see the body after death, and attend the funeral if they wish.

BEREAVEMENT (Parkes 1985; Worden 1991)

Because bereavement due to cancer can usually be foreseen by a matter of months, many relatives have already done some 'anticipatory grieving' beforehand. This is much easier if patient and relative have been able to talk together about the impending death, and agree about practical matters such as the funeral arrangements, the will, and the future care of young children or aged parents.

Another feature of many cancer deaths is a sense of relief. Though this often induces some degree of guilt, it is in fact an appropriate reaction following a long period of suffering which has exhausted both patient and carer:

> *Tina*, age 56, became extremely distressed when her husband was dying from cancer. During the three months of his last illness she developed insomnia, loss of appetite, fear of going out alone, and a marked nervous tremor. Counselling sessions and a course of antidepressants did not help very much, partly because she was so preoccupied with fears regarding the death itself. She had never seen a dead body, and this prospect was repulsive to her. Also she was convinced she could not cope with life on her own.
>
> When the death happened, however, Tina's calm acceptance surprised everyone. She voluntarily helped the nurses to lay out her husband's body, then asked to be left alone with him 'to say goodbye'. She made all the funeral arrangements unaided. Two weeks later all her depressive symptoms had resolved. She said 'Of course I miss him, but it was a happy release for both of us and now I need to build up my own life again.' She remained well six months later.

The Death Itself

Most cancer deaths occur gradually. The patient grows weaker, and stops eating and drinking. He or she may seem withdrawn and show little response to relatives' presence, which may distress them unless they understand it as a natural prelude to the death. Many patients lapse into unconsciousness for a day or two before they actually die.

Less often, death comes unexpectedly suddenly due to some acute complication such as a large haemorrhage from the tumour.

Many relatives will wish to be present when death occurs, and/or to see the body afterwards. Seeing the body is encouraged nowadays, because it appears to promote better longterm emotional adjustment to bereavement, but should never be forced upon relatives who are reluctant.

If the patient is in hospital, news that the patient is dying, or has already died, is best conveyed by a doctor or nurse already known to the family. Too much 'prettifying' of the body before the relatives are allowed to view is not necessarily welcome though judgement is obviously required; for example it makes sense to clear away any vomit or blood. Afterwards, relatives should be offered the opportunity to stay alone with the body for a while.

Though most cancer deaths are to some extent expected, the mode and timing of death can never be predicted with confidence. Relatives may be distressed if the patient dies sooner than anticipated, or if the terminal event was sudden and messy rather than a gradual peaceful decline. Truthful explanation about anything untoward is almost always best, and will minimise any resentment towards the staff involved.

Witnessing another's death may have a powerful effect on patients in hospital. It is often perceived as a comforting experience rather than a distressing one. Distress may, however, result if the death is less than peaceful. Also, while one death may have positive effects, witnessing a whole series of deaths—as often happens for patients who spend long periods in a hospice setting—may become demoralising.

Relatives sometimes like to return to the ward on which their loved one died. As a way of helping to round off the experience, thank the staff and say goodbye, one or two such visits are often mutually rewarding. More than this should not be encouraged because, apart from being likely to interfere with the ongoing work of the ward, repeated visits may indicate a psychological need which would be better met elsewhere. Most hospices offer a formal programme of bereavement support. If this is unavailable, relatives may be given details of voluntary organisations such as CRUSE, or advised to consult the primary care team.

Bereavement Reactions

Much current knowledge about the aftermath of bereavement due to cancer comes from the work of Colin Murray Parkes in London.

The classic sequence of emotional reactions follows four stages, similar to those described in relation to initial diagnosis of cancer:

1. Shock, numbness, disbelief.
2. Acute distress, anger and protest; searching for the dead person.

3. Depression and despair.
4. Acceptance and resolution.

As already discussed, this type of model provides a useful framework but should not be taken too rigidly as many bereavement reactions do not follow such a neat sequence. The picture depends on such factors as the personality of the survivor, the circumstances of the death, availability of social support, and the nature and quality of the relationship with the deceased. Most bereavement research has been carried out on widows; reactions for widowers may be rather different, whereas special issues certainly apply for other groups such as parents who have lost a child, or those in homosexual partnerships.

A bewildering variety of psychological responses may be seen in the aftermath of a loved one's death.

Besides the obvious emotions of sadness, tearfulness and yearning in the first few days or weeks, there may be intense anger or guilt, and sometimes paradoxical feelings like triumph or euphoria. Changes in sleep, appetite and activity are common. A few sleeping tablets or anxiolytics may be a great help at this time, but too much medication may block the grieving process and perhaps create dependence.

It may be a long time before the bereaved person can fully realise the loss. Seeming to see the deceased in a crowd, to hear his or her voice ('pseudohallucinations'), or continuing to set the table for two instead of one, are common experiences; but survivors who are unprepared for them may fear that they are going mad.

William Worden describes 'four tasks of mourning':

1. Accepting the reality of the loss.
2. Experiencing the pain of grief: emotional and vegetative symptoms.
3. Adjusting to an environment without the deceased.
4. Withdrawing emotional energy: reinvestment in new relationships.

Working through all these 'tasks' will take at least a year, or considerably longer in the case of many close relationships. It may indeed be both inappropriate and offensive to suggest that a bereaved person will ever 'get over' his or her loss in the sense of forgetting about the dead person and returning to being the same as before. Many will have been irrevocably changed by their experience and would not wish it otherwise. Despite the pain of the bereavement, they feel themselves strengthened by it. Gradually they become able to take up new relationships and activities again. Christmas and anniversaries, however, may continue to be painful times.

Bereavement is bound to be distressing in almost all circumstances, and longterm adjustment seems to be better when the pain of grief is acknowledged and expressed, rather than artificially suppressed by tranquillisers or a 'stiff upper lip' response. Just as the pain from a physical wound has a protective function, guarding against use of the injured body part before healing has taken place, grief does serve some useful purpose. It is therefore unfortunate that bereavement, despite being a normal experience which occurs during almost every lifetime, is a somewhat taboo subject in modern British society. Open or prolonged expression of grief is not encouraged; people tend to avoid the bereaved, embarrassed by their grief and uncertain what to say; and expressions of emotional support or practical help are often limited to the first week or so, perhaps disappearing before the worst of the grief has even begun.

Sometimes the grieving process 'goes wrong'. This is especially likely after sudden or violent deaths, including suicides; after the untimely deaths of young adults or children; when the relationship between survivor and deceased was ambivalent or dependent; when the survivor lacks a good supportive network, has a vulnerable personality, or a tendency towards alcohol abuse. Variants of abnormal grieving include:

Inhibited grief: avoiding painful emotions by constantly keeping busy, moving away to a new area, premature 'replacement' of a dead spouse by remarriage or a dead child by a new pregnancy. This apparently works for some people, but in others is associated with chronic mild depression, numbness of emotion, or intense sadness triggered by other more trivial losses.

Occasionally there is a complete inability to accept the reality of the death; an extreme form of denial in which the survivor seems to believe that the deceased is still alive. This phenomenon is very rare, and may be associated with low intelligence and/or mental illness.

Daisy, a 60-year-old housewife who had received psychiatric treatment for 'paranoid psychosis' in the past, had been widowed for three months but told people that her husband was in hospital. She had refused to attend his funeral, and claimed his death certificate was a forgery. Daisy's increasing neglect of herself and her home, and verbal abuse of her neighbours, resulted in her compulsory admission to a psychiatric ward. Treatment with a combination of antipsychotic drugs, repeated discussion about her husband, and social rehabilitation had good results, and after discharge home she was able to look afer herself, and to accept her widowed state.

Chronic grief: inability to relinquish the dead person. His or her possessions are carefully kept, with one or more rooms in the house often preserved as a 'shrine'. Direct contact may be sought through spiritualism. The survivor's desire to remain true to the memory of the deceased may rule out a move to a more easily-run house or cultivation of a new relationship. Underlying the idealisation of the dead person may be unacknowledged anger or guilt.

Psychiatric illness is diagnosed in about 20% of widow(ers) followed up in the year after bereavement. The most usual diagnosis is depressive illness; however, it is not always easy to distinguish this from severe grief. Any other type of psychiatric illness, in predisposed people, can be triggered off by the stress of bereavement, and specific psychiatric treatments will be required in addition to bereavement counselling.

Physical illness becomes more common after a bereavement, and death rates in the first year of widow(er)hood are increased. Cardiovascular disorders, suicides and accidents, infectious diseases and cirrhosis of the liver are the main conditions involved (there is *no* evidence to support the popular belief that cancer rates are increased). The discovery of changes in immune function in recently bereaved people has aroused much interest and could provide a direct explanation for some of this increased morbidity. Probably, however, the main explanations lie in the tendency of some bereaved people to drink and smoke more than usual, neglect their diet and become accident-prone. Along with their increased risk of genuine physical illness, the bereaved have an increased tendency to worry about their own health, and may develop hypochondriacal fears centred on the same disease from which their loved one died.

Bereavement Counselling

Most bereaved people adjust through the resources of their own personality and the support of family and friends. Not all of them need specialised help, indeed this might sometimes have the undesirable effects of undermining their own pefectly adequate coping mechanisms, and 'medicalising' an experience which, though painful, is a natural part of life. For the minority at high risk of poor adjustment, counselling can improve the longterm outcome. The aims of bereavement counselling include:

- Helping the survivor to accept the reality of the loss.
- Enabling feelings about the dead person—both positive and negative ones—to be acknowledged and expressed.
- Providing continued support during the period of grieving.
- Providing reassurance about responses which, though disconcerting for the sufferer, fall within the normal range (eg pseudohallucinations).
- Identifying responses which are unhelpful (eg alcohol abuse) or require specialised treatment (eg depressive illness).
- Eventually, facilitating emotional withdrawal from the dead person and adaptation to a new lifestyle.

Talking about the death itself, and about the person who has died, will obviously take up a large part of such counselling sessions. Many clients gain therapeutic benefit from talking through the same material on several occasions. There is, however, some risk of getting stuck in non-productive repetition. This may happen because the facts alone are being discussed without the accompanying emotion—especially if that emotion is of a potentially unacceptable kind, for example anger towards the dead person or relief about the death. The counsellor must win the client's trust in order to release such disclosures, which can be encouraged by a question like 'Is there anything you *won't* miss about X?' Practical techniques may be used, for example bringing old family photographs to facilitate the revival of memories about the deceased—again, it may take time for the less positive memories to come to light—or encouraging the client to visit the grave. Giving direct advice is seldom wise, but the counsellor may wish to encourage some kinds of behaviour and sound a note of caution about others. Some clients seem to need permission to bring their mourning to an end and say a final goodbye. Special techniques such as role-play or letter-writing, designed to express what could never be said to the person who died, can produce a powerful emotional catharsis and should only be used by trained therapists.

The following case history illustrates the use of counselling after bereavement:

Bill, a bachelor in his 40s, had lived all his life with his widowed mother. Each had their strictly-defined roles, Bill going out to work and looking after the car while his mother kept house. When the mother was found to have advanced cancer she had to be admitted to a palliative care ward because Bill, who had never done any domestic work at all, could not begin to manage her care at home.

Bill said 'I've got no future without Mother' and 'There's no point in anything—I won't have her messed about with—all we want is a pill to finish the pair of us off.' He spent all his waking hours at his mother's bedside, crying and stroking her hand. He was identified as at high risk of clinical depression, self-neglect and perhaps deliberate self-harm in his bereavement. The ward staff tried hard to encourage him to talk about his feelings, and also to carry out simple aspects of his mother's physical care, but he resisted all their efforts. His family doctor, who commented that Bill had always been a 'dependent personality', had already tried him on antidepressants with no effect.

continued

continued

After his mother died, Bill accepted weekly home visits from a bereavement counsellor who reported that the house was like a memorial, with photographs of the mother in every room, and her personal things left exactly as they were on the day she was taken to hospital.

Bill remained sunk in despair for many weeks and often greeted the counsellor with wry reference to his suicidal ideas ('Did you bring my cyanide pills this time?'). He described his mother in idealised terms as a paragon of beauty, virtue and domestic industry.

Gradually, over many months, changes became evident. Bill started to do more things around the house, and would take a child-like pride in presenting the counsellor with a cup of tea he had made, or showing her the newly-washed kitchen floor. He continued to idealise his mother but also began to reveal some resentment of the strict control she had exercised over his life. One Saturday he went to a football match, which he had seldom been allowed to do during her lifetime. As the first anniversary of her death approached his despair returned, and on the day itself he got drunk, but after that seemed to improve.

The counsellor had been well aware from the start that Bill might develop a strong dependency on her also, and that she would have to set firm limits on the relationship at the same time as providing consistent longterm support. For example, she stood by the initial arrangement of visiting once a week although Bill often asked her to increase it to twice a week; and while accepting his cups of tea, she politely declined his offer of a meal to show off his newfound cooking skills. Very slowly, besides becoming more self-sufficient in the home, Bill began to take up some hobbies and social life, and he packed up some of his mother's clothes for a local charity shop. Although it seemed unlikely that he would ever completely resolve the grieving process, after eighteen months his adjustment seemed sufficiently secure for the counsellor to taper off her visits. About this time, Bill revealed that he had met a new woman friend.

FURTHER READING

Auchincloss S. Sexual dysfunction in cancer patients. In Holland JC, Rowland JH (eds) (1989) *Handbook of Psychooncology*. Oxford University Press: New York

Couldrick A (1988) *Grief and bereavement: understanding children* and Couldrick A (1991). *When your mum or dad has cancer.* Booklets available from: Sobell Publications, Sir Michael Sobell House, Churchill Hospital, Oxford OX3 7LJ

Parkes, CM (1985) Bereavement. *British Journal of Psychiatry 146* 11–17

Rait D, Lederberg MS. The family of the cancer patient. In Holland JC, Rowland JH (eds) (1989) *Handbook of Psychooncology.* Oxford University Press: New York

Smith N, Regnard C (1993) Managing family problems in advanced disease—a flow diagram. *Palliative Medicine 7* 47–58

Worden W (1991) *Grief Counselling and Grief Therapy.* London: Routledge

6
Issues for Oncology Staff

The topics covered in this section include: how to break bad news and respond to awkward questions, why some patients evoke strong feelings in the staff who care for them, and the prevention and management of emotional problems among staff themselves.

These are not specialised topics—they form an integral part of day-to-day clinical practice. Some staff, finding the technical aspects of oncology more interesting and less threatening than the psychosocial ones, like to believe they can ignore the kind of issues discussed here. They are mistaken. Every staff–patient interaction is bound to contain personal aspects which, whether or not they are consciously recognised, may have lasting emotional consequences for either or both of the people concerned.

TALKING WITH PATIENTS ABOUT CANCER (Brewin 1991; Maguire 1985)

This section begins with some recommendations about how to conduct a planned 'bad news consultation', then continues with discussion of how to handle some of the awkward questions which patients may ask at unexpected times.

Some doctors and nurses find these issues so difficult that they become adept at avoiding them. Ways of doing this include: focusing entirely on physical symptoms, advising the patient to put their questions to someone else instead, or keeping away from the patient altogether. By using such strategies they are neglecting an important aspect of their work.

The skill of talking with patients about cancer comes easier to some staff than others but can to some extent be learned. The following list of 'do's' and 'don't's' for conducting interviews may help.

Do:
- Allow time.
- Ensure privacy.
- Respect confidentiality.
- Let the patient talk.
- Listen to what the patient says.
- Be sensitive to 'non-verbal cues' such as facial expression.
- Gauge the need for information on an individual basis.
- Permit painful topics.
- Permit silences.

Don't:
- Assume you know what is troubling the patient.
- Give false reassurance.
- Overload with information.
- Feel obliged to keep talking all the time.
- Withhold information.
- Tell lies.
- Criticise or make judgements.
- Give direct advice about psychological matters.

There are no rules about what choice of words, facial expression and tone of voice are correct; it depends on the patient's case, and the personality of the staff member. The use of humour, for example, might be the key to success in one clinical interview, but a disaster in another (and is best avoided in the case of doubt).

Breaking Bad News

At one time, concealing a diagnosis of cancer from patients themselves was common practice, although the truth might be revealed to the relatives—often placing a heavy burden of secrecy or deception upon them. The same convention still holds in some parts of the world, including many southern and eastern European countries. Nowadays in the UK, as in the rest of northern Europe and North America, almost all cancer patients are told what is wrong. Many of them continue to feel they have been kept in the dark about the details of their illness, and perceive various shortfalls in communication with their doctors. This may not be entirely the doctors' fault because, during emotionally-charged interviews, patients often forget what questions they wanted to ask, or dare not ask them, or fail to take in what they are told. The flourishing of such organisations as BACUP and Cancer Link (page 158) attests to the hunger for information felt by many cancer patients and their families today.

A few patients complain of being told too much; this often reflects tactlessness or poor timing in the way information was given. It could also be that the pendulum has swung too far away from the old-style secrecy about cancer, so that complete stark truthfulness is seen as essential and patients are not allowed to use denial as a mental defence.

Breaking bad news—conveying the initial diagnosis of cancer, explaining that a recurrence has developed or that X-ray appearances are worse in spite of treatment—can seem a daunting task. It may be helpful to remember that most patients find uncertainty, which is often accompanied by anxiety and morbid fantasies, harder to bear than knowing the facts.

Who should break the news? An experienced doctor, who already knows the patient and is going to be involved in future clinical care, is usually the best person. Whether this should be a hospital consultant / senior registrar or the patient's own family doctor is sometimes open to discussion. The rank and status of the person concerned is, however, less important than whether he or she is well-informed and empathic. Very often in hospital settings, it is the more junior doctors and nurses who find themselves faced with direct questions from patients, or with requests to explain what the consultant has already said.

Learning bad news by accident—overhearing a conversation on the ward round (bedside curtains are not sound-proof!), or from a chance remark by a staff member who assumes the patient already knew—usually causes distress. Bad news is best conveyed in a planned fashion if this is possible.

The practical setting is important. Choose a private room, allow adequate time and guard against interruptions. Do not have a large retinue present—two or three staff is the maximum. The patient, if well enough, should be allowed the dignity of being up and dressed and sitting on the same physical level as the doctor. A close relative or friend may provide valuable support, but whether to have such a person present or not is the patient's decision. The practice of telling the spouse or close relative but not the patient largely belongs in the past, and can only be justified for patients too young, too old or too ill to understand for themselves.

Brutal frankness of the 'you've got cancer and we can't chop it out so we're sending you home tomorrow' variety causes needless distress to patients. The opposite tactic of using vague euphemisms and skirting around the facts is also unsatisfactory, because it may leave patients feeling patronised or perplexed. Plain language sympathetically spoken is best. Though the word 'cancer' may indeed evoke fear and stigma, talk of 'a growth' or 'a tumour' or 'nasty cells' or 'not a very nice lump' can be mystifying, and most patients find it easier if 'cancer' is openly named.

How much detailed information is given about various aspects of the illness should be guided by the progress of the interview, the doctor being sensitive to verbal and non-verbal cues from the patient. Some patients want to know much more than others, and it may be best to ask directly 'Do you want me to explain any further?' at various points. Do not make assumptions about which concerns are most important. Many patients have an obvious fear such as dying in pain—others may be worrying about something quite different, such as family finances or the welfare of a pet.

However bad the news, it is most important to offer some positive messages, always providing these are truthful ones. Make it clear that help with pain control or the care of a frail spouse will be available, and that the patient will never be abandoned although there may come a time when active anticancer treatment will be stopped.

Not everything can be taken in at once. Patients may need information repeated on several occasions, even if detailed explanations have already been given. Written leaflets are very useful in the case of standardised treatments. In a few clinics, the consultation is recorded on audiotape for the patient to take home, and research studies suggest that most patients appreciate this.

Emotional displays of tears or anger should be permitted, even if some staff find them embarrassing. On occasion, patients' anger about their illness is projected towards the person who told them the bad news—the 'shoot the messenger' response—which can be hurtful to staff who did their best. Just listening, without self-righteous defence or getting angry back, is usually the best way to deal with this. Many patients will realise later on what has happened, and apologise.

Sometimes staff themselves will be upset during the interview. There is no need to conceal this at all costs. Extreme professional detachment, in which the doctor or nurse comes over as an unfeeling robot, is not welcome to most patients. They prefer some evidence of human warmth, and may find it comforting to see that staff are emotionally affected by the bad news too. Obviously, however, some moderation is called for. It is not advisable for staff to break down completely in front of their patients, nor to pour out details of their own personal sorrows.

It is most important that some followup contact, preferably with the same person who conveyed the bad news, is offered after a 'bad news consultation'.

In some cases, a single formal interview of the type described above is not appropriate for various reasons. The bad news may have become gradually apparent and been broken in stages. Some patients, using denial, seem to avoid wanting to hear it and this raises the issue of how far the staff should try to persuade them to talk. Probably the best way is to give repeated clear opportunities for the patient to ask questions:

Patient dying of lung cancer: 'I'll soon be over this chest infection—I want to get home for Christmas."
Doctor or nurse: 'We all hope you will, but have you ever thought you might not be well enough to go?"

This leaves the options open for the patient. If he says 'No way, I'll be right as rain by then' he is giving a clear message that further questions are unwelcome and this should be respected. If he says

'Well, I try to look on the positive side but I do wonder if I'll ever get home again' the doctor or nurse could go further: 'You wonder if you're going to get better from this illness?"

Responding to Awkward Questions

Questions like 'Am I going to get better?' or 'How long have I got?' are natural enough, but are sometimes asked quite suddenly out of the blue and catch the doctor or nurse unawares.

Many patients given a diagnosis of cancer will want to know details of their prognosis; what is the likelihood of cure and, if cure is not possible, how much longer they can expect to live. Without answers to such questions, it is difficult to make either practical decisions or psychological adjustments.

However, there is seldom any accurate way of predicting the future in an individual case. Statistical generalisations can be given (for example '50% of patients with your type of cancer will still be alive after five years'), but are not always helpful, especially for the less well educated. Many patients find this lack of precision hard to understand or accept, and may feel their doctors are deliberately hiding the truth if they give a vague prognosis. Doctors, in turn, often feel pressurised to provide an answer and may hazard a guess: 'perhaps six months or so'. Naming an exact time span like this, however tentative the phrasing, often proves a mistake because six months ahead becomes fixed as a crucial date in the minds of both patient and family. If death comes sooner, completion of important tasks may have been put off too long, and the relatives feel cheated. If on the other hand the patient survives the deadline, it may be with an uneasy feeling of living on borrowed time, and with regrets over premature decisions hurriedly made. Saying 'probably months rather than years' or 'weeks rather than months' is often as precise as it is wise to be.

Prognostic uncertainty is, for many patients, one of the hardest aspects of having cancer. Staff have to acknowledge this, rather than make unfounded predictions which make them (though not necessarily the patient) feel better in the short term at the risk of causing problems later on. It may be worth pointing out that life expectancy is not known for anyone—a perfectly healthy person might die tomorrow in a car crash—and that everybody, cancer patient or not, is well advised to make the most of the present day.

Other awkward questions relate to the mode of dying: 'How am I going to die?' Some patients are afraid of choking or bleeding to death, often because they have seen this happen to another patient in the ward or to one of their own relatives in the past. Although a gradual, peaceful and pain-free death can be achieved for many, this cannot be guaranteed for all, and it would be dishonest to make firm promises. One can only listen to the patient's fears, and explain that they are unlikely to materialise but say what could be done to ease distress if they did.

Remember that blunt direct questions do not always call for cut-and-dried answers, but for some patients are a way of indicating that they would like to discuss their concerns more generally. It is sometimes best to answer with another question: 'Would you like to say a bit more about that?' or 'I wonder if you had any special reason for asking?' It can be vital to clarify what the question really means before providing a specific reply. A young businesswoman with advanced breast cancer asked 'How much longer do you think it will be?' The doctor assumed she was asking how long she had to live, but fortunately realised just in time that she meant 'How long before I can get out of hospital and go back to work?' Otherwise, abruptly shattering her defence of denial might have provoked great distress.

Criticisms of Colleagues

Nearly all patients, by the time they arrive at a specialised cancer treatment unit, have been under the care of their family doctor and perhaps other hospital departments. It is not unusual for them to make criticisms, direct or indirect, about their previous care, and some ask questions like 'If Dr X had referred me here to start with, could I have been cured?' It is all too easy to collude with blaming Dr X without knowing the circumstances at the time. On the other hand, there are clearly cases in which the diagnosis was unduly delayed or treatment mishandled, and it would seem wrong to close professional ranks and automatically defend one's colleagues. Giving a clear verdict as to whether or not Dr X was at fault is seldom the best way to respond. Listen to the patient's point of view and, if a frank complaint is involved, perhaps suggest a direct approach to the doctor concerned.

'SPECIAL' PATIENTS (Grant 1980; Lederberg 1989a)

'Special' patients may appear to fall into two opposite categories—the unusually likeable or interesting ones who attract overinvolvement from staff, and the unpopular ones whom staff find difficult and unrewarding. These two categories are not so different as they seem.

Although the heading of this section refers to *patients*, much of the following material applies equally to *staff*. It is all too easy, in healthcare settings where professionals have the upper hand, to put the blame for any problems entirely on the patients' side.

Overinvolvement with Patients

Some idealistic doctors and nurses might question whether it is ever possible to be overinvolved with patients—but most would probably agree that taking too close an interest is undesirable.

Signs of overinvolvement include spending unusually long periods of time with the patients concerned; granting them extra privileges such as phone calls or appointments outside normal working hours; assuming responsibility for other aspects of their lives besides their illness; thinking about them frequently outside the work setting; and relaxing the usual professional boundaries so that social or even sexual contact develops.

What leads to overinvolvement? It may result from 'identification' in cases where the patient's age and sex, personality and circumstances are rather similar to the staff member's own; or from a 'transference' phenomenon in which the patient evokes unconscious memories of an important figure from the staff member's past. Patients who themselves have a medical or nursing background often attract overinvolvement. In other cases, it happens because the staff member concerned—usually a doctor in this instance—has a strong investment in the mode of treatment being used; perhaps a promising new drug being tested in a clinical trial. Lastly, overinvolvement with patients may reflect a lack of satisfying close relationships in the staff member's own personal life.

Sometimes the extra staff efforts do pay worthwhile dividends, so the patient makes a good response to treatment and shows due appreciation for all that has been done. But apart from leading to an unfair allocation of care—extra time spent with the 'special' patient means less attention for 'ordinary' ones— overinvolvement may lead to an intense relationship between patient and staff member which is almost bound to build up unrealistic expectations, and sometimes goes badly wrong.

Dr A, a consultant oncologist, devoted huge efforts to the case of a young woman, a general practitioner's wife, who had advanced breast cancer. He carried out all aspects of her medical care in person, whereas with most similar cases he would probably have delegated some aspects to his junior staff and also liaised with colleagues in the palliative care unit. Like many doctors' relatives, the patient was not registered with a GP of her own.

When the patient was dying at home, Dr A visited most evenings and told her husband 'Call me any time, day or night.' Both patient and husband were very grateful for Dr A's attentions.

Her condition remained stable for several weeks, perhaps rather longer than anticipated, and when Dr A's own wife persuaded him to take her to Paris for the weekend of their wedding anniversary he thought his patient would be alright for a couple of days. That Saturday night, however, the patient developed spinal cord compression. Her husband made repeated phone calls to Dr A's home but got no reply. He eventually obtained help through the hospital but with some difficulty because nobody else was familiar with the case and the notes, it seemed, were in Dr A's briefcase.

The patient was deeply distressed by what she perceived as Dr A's desertion, sobbing 'He wasn't there when we needed him' and asked to be transferred to another consultant. The husband tried to patch things up with Dr A, saying 'Can't be helped—just one of those things', but seemed somewhat embarrassed and displeased. The couple never recovered their close relationship with Dr A, who was left feeling guilty and puzzled about the matter.

The 'Difficult' Patient

Some patients inspire negative reactions such as irritation, anger, guilt or despair in the doctors and nurses looking after them. The various reasons for this may be grouped as follows:

- *Patients with 'difficult' personalities*: the problem is a chronic one, which reflects ingrained attitudes and behaviour. This has often been written about from the primary care perspective, because it is general practitioners who bear the brunt of coping with these patients over many years. Such patients frequently attend the doctor's surgery with trivial minor illnesses or hypochondriacal complaints. Their medical and social backgrounds are complex and some have 'secrets' such as sexual abuse in childhood. Despite their frequent demands for medical attention, they often refuse or indirectly sabotage the advice given, and seem to have a knack of setting up conflicts between the various professionals involved in their care. Not surprisingly, they evoke strong negative feelings in these professionals, as reflected in such vivid but disparaging labels as 'hateful', 'heartsink' or 'fat-file' patient. In psychiatric terminology, many of them have chronic somatisation disorder. If and when such patients develop cancer, their management may continue to pose difficulties; though it may also happen that, under the stress of a genuine life-threatening illness, new dignity and maturity emerge.
- *Patients undergoing atypical adjustment reactions*: some people, normally perfectly pleasant and reasonable, react to the stress of their current illness by developing 'difficult' behaviour. They may be openly rude and angry; or give the impression of sulky resentment; or appear flat and unmotivated despite all the treatment efforts being made on their behalf. Applying the dismissive 'heartsink' label may make the staff feel better for a while, but is all too often an excuse to give up any genuine effort to help. Underneath, most such patients are very frightened and unhappy, and some are clinically depressed. Continued provision of understanding and care, attention to symptom control such as relief of pain combined with psychotropic drug therapy if indicated, may eventually bring good results.
- *Patients being 'scapegoated' for other problems*: some patients get labelled 'difficult' for reasons which are most unfair. This can

happen when the personal problems of staff, or the shortfalls of the healthcare system, get displaced onto the work setting as in the following examples. A nurse, irritable because her child had refused to go to bed before she came on night duty, scolded a patient who could not go to sleep. A doctor who was having trouble putting up a drip on a man whose veins were blocked from previous chemotherapy told him crossly 'You really are an awful nuisance.' An elderly patient, having to wait several weeks for a place in a longstay ward, was criticised for blocking an acute bed. In other cases, it is the relatives who are difficult but the patient who is blamed.

Management: the essential first steps involve acknowledging the problem and considering what lies behind it. These may be hard steps to take. Some staff are very ready to call their patients difficult, but less willing to concede that they themselves are playing any part in the conflict. Others, for whom any negative feelings towards patients go against their code of professional ethics, cannot admit such problems to their colleagues nor perhaps even privately to themselves. This is particularly true in hospice settings, where staff may aspire to be paragons of virtue! If the feelings are not acknowledged, further problems may follow. The patient in question may be covertly punished, for example by prescription of an unpleasant treatment, or premature discharge from followup. Alternatively, the negative feelings are displaced onto another patient, a (usually junior) colleague, or the staff member's family; or the staff member develops signs of 'burnout'.

Once the problem is out in the open it may become possible to make a fresh start. Simply talking over the issues can help. If the problem is specific to one member of staff, who for whatever reason has a personality clash with a particular patient, discussion with a detached professional colleague may suggest ways to improve matters; if not, a change of doctor or nurse may be best. More often, the difficulties are shared by a number of people. It may then be useful to arrange a case conference which includes the primary care team as well as hospital staff, and perhaps the patient and family too.

It is most important to decide on a consistent approach which is agreed between everyone concerned, including the patient.

Setting specific practical goals, in writing, is usually helpful. Similarly it is often useful to agree clear limits, for example regarding the frequency and duration of consultations. Progress on both counts can be recorded in diary form.

The aims should not be too ambitious, if the problems are longstanding and deepseated ones. On the other hand there is almost always some scope for improvement. Difficult patients benefit from understanding and care just as much as any other patients do, even if it tries the patience of staff to provide this. Patients can usually tell if staff dislike them or have given up on their case, and will often react by becoming more difficult still.

As many different professionals are likely to be involved, it is useful to be clear about who is responsible for which specific aspects of the case, and for one senior named doctor to be in overall charge.

The 'Special' Patient

Sometimes, when patients who were initially perceived as unusually interesting and attractive fail to get better, their image undergoes a subtle change so that staff come to regard them as 'difficult' instead. It is as if they are paying the price for not responding to all the effort put into their case, or for making the overinvolved staff member feel sheepish when he or she realises what has happened. Probably less often the reverse occurs—a 'difficult' patient makes a positive response to good professional care and the staff gradually find themselves getting fond of that patient after all.

It would be impossible to like all patients equally, or give every one the same amount of attention. Patients who inspire strong feelings, whether positive or negative, add variety to working life. Only by recognising these strong feelings can they be harnessed in a constructive fashion.

PERSONAL SUPPORT: AVOIDING 'BURNOUT'
(Alexander 1993; Lederberg 1989b;
Riordan and Saltzer 1992)

All branches of medicine and nursing are in some respects stressful. In any specialty, stressful aspects are likely to outweigh rewarding ones if practical conditions are poor, if the right kind of support for staff is not available, or if the staff members concerned are temperamentally unsuited to working in the field. When these factors apply, the strikingly-named though loosely-defined syndrome of 'burnout' may arise.

Burnout

This syndrome develops when the demands on staff exceed their resources. Early signs include tiredness, irritability, poor concentration, and physical symptoms such as headache or backache—such responses to stress at work are extremely common and in many cases they recover after a bad patch is over, or with the help of a few days off. Sometimes, however, they progress to a more chronic and deep-seated problem. The classic pattern is one of growing boredom and cynicism, in which case the affected staff member may arrive late and leave early, cut corners at work, and behave in off-hand fashion towards both patients and colleagues.

Less often, the picture is one of obsessive dedication to the job ("Messiah syndrome"), leading to neglect of personal and family life, punishing schedules for junior colleagues, and progressive exhaustion. The situation may drag on till retirement, often with less and less insight on the part of the person concerned, or may result in a crisis: abuse of alcohol or drugs, major depression, attempted or completed suicide.

Burnout is probably more common in some work settings than others, whether because the work is intrinsically more stressful, or because staff with certain personality characteristics are attracted to such work. Different specialties carry different types of stress. Many studies have focused on oncology nurses, for whom two particular issues are having to give their patients drugs which make them feel very ill, and seeing a high proportion of their patients—including many young ones—deteriorate and die.

When Patients Die

Although cancer is by no means always fatal, death is a fairly commonplace event in cancer treatment units. Most of these deaths, being an inevitable outcome of the illness, are accepted as predictable and timely. Their impact upon the staff therefore is rather different from that of deaths in certain other hospital settings. Unlike, say, the death of a young woman in childbirth or the suicide of a patient on a psychiatric ward, deaths from cancer seldom precipitate intense shock, distress or guilt. Even so, cancer deaths do have emotional effects on the staff, especially on the nurses who have provided close care towards the end of life and perhaps become very fond of the patient and family. Dealing with many deaths in close succession also takes a toll.

Even after years of experience, a doctor or nurse may feel personal grief when a patient dies. This is especially likely when 'identification' with that patient was present. Sometimes it has parallels with a bereavement in the staff member's own personal life. A more complicated reaction may ensue if the staff member feels at fault in any way—for example, having given medication which probably hastened the death, or failed to call the relatives in time.

Traditionally, professionals have been trained to suppress their own feelings in this situation. Some degree of emotional detachment is indeed required for people working in this field, otherwise they would soon be overwhelmed by sadness, but when it goes too far the result is the cynical callous attitude of the burnout syndrome.

Maintaining Staff Morale

The following suggestions may be helpful, and apply to the most senior personnel as well as to younger doctors and nurses:

- Staff selection: highly dedicated, idealistic people have much to offer but may be at particular risk.
- Work conditions: avoidance of excessive hours and excessive caseloads, pleasant physical surroundings.
- Informal staff interaction: spontaneous discussions over coffee often do more good than official 'support' sessions. Humour, including the black variety, can be a valuable form of emotional release but also has the potential to offend.
- Formal staff support: encouraging a team spirit and shared objectives, availability of individual counselling, and staff

support groups. Groups run on psychotherapeutic lines are not necessarily helpful and may sometimes be damaging, for example when members feel under pressure to attend, or to reveal personal material to their colleagues. Groups with an educational theme are often less threatening and more constructive.

- Encouraging self-care: time off, enough sleep, good diet, restraint in use of drugs including alcohol and tobacco, personal relationships and hobbies outside work, physical exercise.

Given good support, many staff consider the oncology setting a rewarding one. Interest in the scientific or technical aspects is of course important. On a more personal level, many staff find satisfaction and a sense of privilege from accompanying patients and families through such a major transition in their lives, and witnessing the strength with which so many weather this.

Some people, however, are fundamentally unsuited for working with cancer patients. This is no cause for shame and should be acknowledged as early as possible for everyone's benefit. They will almost certainly be able to find another branch of nursing or medicine, better suited to their individual qualities, in which they can achieve greater personal satisfaction and therefore contribute more to patient care.

FURTHER READING

Alexander DA (1993) Staff support groups: do they support and are they even groups? *Palliative Medicine 7* 127–32

Brewin TB (1991) Three ways of giving bad news. *Lancet 337* 1207–9

Grant WB (1980). The hated patient and his hating attendants. *Medical Journal of Australia* (volume 2 for 67th year; July) 727–9

Lederberg MS. The confluence of psychiatry, the law and ethics. In Holland JC, Rowland JH (eds) (1989a) *Handbook of Psychooncology*. Oxford University Press: New York

Lederberg MS. Psychological problems of staff and their management. In Holland JC, Rowland JH (eds) (1989b) *Handbook of Psychooncology*. Oxford University Press: New York

Maguire P (1985) Psychological barriers to the care of the dying. *British Medical Journal 291* 1711–3

Riordan RJ, Saltzer SK (1992) Burnout prevention among health care providers working with the terminally ill: a literature review. *Omega 25* 17–24

7
Specialised Treatments in Psycho-oncology

Many of the techniques used in mental healthcare settings can be applied to the treatment of emotional problems in cancer patients. They also have a role in the management of cancer pain. Such techniques are complex, and so is the terminology to describe them. An outline of some selected psychological therapies and psychotropic drugs is given here.

This section is not intended as a do-it-yourself manual. The methods described should only be applied by those with specialised training in one of the mental healthcare professions, or else under close supervision by such a specialist. In amateur hands, these techniques may do more harm than good.

Just as oncology staff need education in the use of psychological treatments, however, so mental healthcare professionals need preparation for working in oncology. They should become familiar with the normal spectrum of emotional responses to cancer; with the organic brain syndromes sometimes caused by cancer and its treatment; and with the culture of the hospital unit concerned.

Having cancer is virtually always distressing to some extent. It is not possible, nor would it be appropriate, to abolish this distress completely with psychotherapy or psychotropic drugs. However, skilful use of these treatments either alone or in combination can often do much to improve patients' emotional wellbeing.

INTRODUCING PSYCHOLOGICAL TREATMENTS: COUNSELLING (Breitbart and Holland 1993; Davis and Fallowfield 1991; Watson 1983, 1991)

Definition of Terms

The words 'counselling' and 'psychotherapy' carry a mystique. 'Psychological therapies', 'non-drug therapies' or 'talking treatments' are alternative terms. Anthony Storr provides a simple definition: 'the art of alleviating personal difficulties through the agency of words and a personal professional relationship'.

'Counselling' and 'psychotherapy' are both umbrella terms, often used rather loosely. While they overlap considerably, 'psychotherapy' is the more formalised and ambitious of the two. 'Counselling' can be employed to help ordinary people come to terms with stressful life situations; in the words of the British Association for Counselling, 'The task of counselling is to give the client an opportunity to explore, discover and clarify ways of living more resourcefully and towards greater wellbeing.' In contrast, 'psychotherapy' is designed to achieve lasting personality change in people with more deepseated and longstanding psychopathology. It follows that counselling may be appropriate for a large number of patients with cancer, and also for their relatives, whereas formal psychotherapy is indicated for a minority only.

The hundreds of different 'schools' of psychotherapy and counselling cannot be described here. However, their similarities are more important than their differences. Whatever theoretical technique is being used, the relationship between therapist and client is crucial to the success—or otherwise—of the procedure. *Counselling for cancer patients* might include the following aims:

- Permit ventilation of feelings.
- Provide practical information about the illness, correct false assumptions and dispel unjustified fears.
- Encourage helpful ways of coping.
- Draw attention to any obvious 'maladaptive' strategies the patient is using, such as trying to keep the diagnosis a secret from everyone, or drinking too much alcohol.
- Provide interest and support, and affirm the patient's self-worth.

Nurse-counsellors

Nurse-counsellors are employed in some cancer treatment units, often specialising in a particular condition such as breast or bowel cancer. Ideally, the nurse-counsellor should be present during the medical consultation when the diagnosis is explained, then spend some time alone with the patient to make sure that information has been correctly understood, and discuss any relevant treatment choices—for example whether a breast cancer patient should undergo a mastectomy or opt for local excision with radiotherapy. The nurse-counsellor continues to follow the patient, and if relevant the main carer, through the proposed course of treatment, offering practical advice—for example on choice of a prosthesis after surgery—combined with psychological support. This may reveal more serious emotional problems which merit discussion with the general practitioner and/or referral to a psychiatrist or psychologist with expertise in the field. Virtually all patients are highly appreciative of support from a good nurse-counsellor.

Peer Group Counselling

Professional counsellors cannot understand the cancer experience in the same way as patients who have been through it themselves. Counselling from a 'veteran' patient may have a powerful influence, often for good but occasionally for harm. Some of the patients who volunteer to take up this work are, without realising it, seeking help for their own problems in adjusting to cancer.

Patient organisations which want to bring their members' expertise into the hospital setting should generally be welcomed, but some form of supervision is desirable to make sure that counselling is not being forced upon those new patients who do not want it, that patients are not being upset by the process, and that the volunteers do not overstep their brief by attempting in-depth psychotherapy. Ideally, some training in counselling technique should be given to these volunteers, and a named mental health professional be available to step in if problems arise.

Private Counselling

Increased patient demand for counselling, which is not always available in NHS settings, has encouraged the setting up of private services for cancer patients. Because private counselling is not regulated, the standard of practitioners varies greatly. The best are both skilled and sincere; the worst are misguided or corrupt. In between are many well-intentioned but ineffective practitioners, who often continue seeing their clients for months or years although there is little real benefit to justify the expenditure of so much money and time.

Efficacy of Counselling and Psychotherapy

Several research studies in which cancer patients are randomly allocated to two groups, one having counselling or psychotherapy and the other not, have been published. Most of them have found that treated patients have a better psychological outcome, and that the intervention has few unwanted effects. There is even preliminary evidence that treated patients may have a longer survival time. Such research studies are often flawed by the fact that those patients with strong views about counselling decline to take part—some are quite clear they do not want it, whereas others are so determined to have it that they will if necessary pay for it elsewhere.

Patient Choice in Therapy

Not all cancer patients want counselling or psychotherapy if this is offered. Still fewer take the initiative in requesting it. Yet some staff in those cancer treatment units which have ready access to a therapist take it upon themselves to make referrals without proper discussion with the patients concerned. This is probably because psychological matters are still widely regarded as stigmatised or embarrassing.

Most patients, even if somewhat taken by surprise to find a psychiatrist, psychologist or counsellor at their bedside, will in fact accept an invitation to talk over the emotional aspects of their illness, and may well feel better after doing so. Tactfully introduced and conducted, and kept at a fairly low-key level, most such preliminary interviews do good rather than harm. Some patients, however, would have preferred to refuse them, were it not for the passivity and deference which goes with being in a hospital bed. Even in the case of a preliminary interview, and certainly if regular therapeutic sessions are proposed, patients should be given a true choice about taking part.

When the patient lacks motivation or is frankly unwilling to cooperate, the therapist can sometimes work indirectly through other staff. Meetings during which staff can share their concerns or frustrations about the patient, consider the reasons which might lie behind the problem, and agree a consistent plan of management with a date for review, can have good results.

PSYCHODYNAMIC THERAPY (Brown and Pedder 1991)

Fullscale use of this longterm and ambitious treatment, which is based on psychoanalysis, is seldom indicated for cancer patients but its briefer and more focused variants can usefully be applied.

The central aim of psychodynamic therapy with cancer patients can in most cases be summed up as enabling the expression and 'working through' of grief about the diagnosis and all the associated losses. This may enable discovery of some personal meaning in the illness, and lead to a sense of mastery over it.

Psychodynamic therapy explores the patient's current problems in the context of his or her remembered past life experiences and relationships with other people. The classic caricature of such therapy—the patient lying on the couch and saying whatever comes to mind while the analyst maintains an impassive silence—does not convey an accurate picture of modern practice. Therapists nowadays play a more active part and, although recounting of material from the past may be important, great emphasis is placed upon what actually takes place within the session between the two people involved. The alternative name, 'interpretive therapy', reflects the therapist's role of helping the patient understand the hidden significance of feelings, behaviours and dreams.

Simple examples of the application of psychodynamic techniques with cancer patients include:

- Linking past and present. An elderly man undergoing cancer treatment recalls his wartime combat; exploring the parallels between these two experiences may achieve a better adjustment to both.
- Interpreting mental defence mechanisms. When a sick husband is irritable towards his wife, both partners may feel better if they realise he is *projecting* his unacknowledged anger and frustration about his condition. When a young woman with cancer turns to her mother rather than her husband, she may be *regressing* under the stress of the illness. In some cases, especially in the case of *denial*, defence mechanisms are serving their purpose of protecting the patient from distress and are better left unchallenged.
- Interpreting the transference and countertransference. The way patient and therapist feel and behave towards one another may mirror their interactions with others outside therapy.
- Identifying resistance. What a patient does *not* choose to discuss may be important.
- Interpreting dreams. Patients' unspoken, unacknowledged fears are often clearly manifest in this way.

Classical psychodynamic therapy consists of regular frequent sessions, once a week or more, continued for at least a year and often considerably longer. Such regimes are usually inappropriate for cancer patients, who need a briefer therapy, with sessions flexibly timed to fit in with other hospital appointments and to allow for fluctuations in wellbeing.

Another difference from psychotherapy with physically healthy people concerns the intensity of the relationship with the therapist, which in psychodynamic work is usually considered a powerful factor in the treatment, but may be diluted for cancer patients who are receiving care from a number of different professionals at the same time. Also, whereas in classical psychodynamic therapy the patient is seen alone, it is often important with cancer patients that the partner is in some way included, perhaps with another therapist if not in the same sessions as the patient.

The issue of patient (client) choice and motivation is of prime importance for psychodynamic work. Benefit is only to be expected for those who actively wish to change certain aspects of their feelings, behaviour, or patterns of relating to other people. Patients should also be aware that psychodynamic therapy can be a painful process, involving the recall of bad memories from the past and facing up to the less admirable aspects of their own personalities.

BEHAVIOUR THERAPY (Mastrovito 1989)

Behaviour therapy developed in the 1950s as an alternative to psychodynamic therapy and as something of a rival to it. While the psychodynamic approach explores the possible origins of patients' symptoms in considerable detail, the behavioural one takes the symptoms at face value, making no attempt to link them with past experience or with underlying beliefs or emotions.

Behaviour therapy uses a structured practical approach to discourage unwanted behaviours and substitute more desirable ones.

Examples of problems which are commonly found among cancer patients, and might be suitably tackled with a behavioural approach, include:

- Inability to look at a mastectomy scar or change a colostomy bag.
- Nausea in anticipation of chemotherapy.
- Fear of being alone under a radiotherapy machine or scanner.
- Reluctance to go out because strangers seem to be staring.
- Pain which gets worse in certain emotional situations.
- Excessive bodily checking for signs of recurrent cancer.

Therapy would begin with listing the problems, and rating the severity of those which can be measured on a simple scale: how bad is the anxiety on a scale of 1 to 10?; how many times a day does the patient check her breast for lumps? Also, making a list of desirable goals: going swimming, visiting a friend. A plan of decreasing the unwanted behaviour, and replacing it with more pleasant and constructive activities, is agreed with the patient. It is usually best to begin with something fairly easy, and enlist a relative's help. A written daily record of progress is made.

Much of this therapy is based on simple commonsense, but some technical terms for the different approaches include:

- Desensitisation: gradual (re)introduction to the feared experience.
- Response prevention: for unwanted practical behaviours.
- Thought stopping: for unwanted recurrent thoughts.
- Modelling: by the therapist, or another patient.
- Distraction: diverting attention from anxiety or pain, either by practical activity, or special techniques such as mental imagery.

Unlike some other types of psychotherapy, behaviour therapy requires little sophistication on the patient's part, and its more basic applications can be used effectively with hospitalised patients who cannot or will not cooperate with an interpretive approach.

Walter, aged 70, had myeloma. Because his intense bouts of pain never occurred when he had visitors, and because they responded so quickly to the arrival of a nurse carrying an injection, staff suspected a psychological element. Although Walter appeared frightened about his illness, he resisted all invitations to talk about his feelings. The nurses became concerned that he was taking up more and more of their time but not getting any better.

Walter's key nurse, in consultation with Walter himself, prepared a timetable to show exactly when his regular drugs would be given, and the frequency of planned nursing visits to his room. Activities which Walter enjoyed—relaxation to music, and craft work—were added to the timetable, as were the ward mealtimes. This left several blank periods in his daily schedule, but none were more than half an hour long, and he agreed he should not normally need to ring the bell during those times but might spend them listening to a tape. He was also asked to keep a written record of the timing and intensity of his pain. Introducing this framework, designed to give Walter more sense of security and active participation in his own care, was followed by an improvement.

The ethical aspects of behavioural regimes should be carefully monitored, especially if the patient is not capable of giving informed consent to them. The use of 'rewards' to encourage the desired behaviour can too easily become extended to include punishments also.

Other techniques often combined with behaviour therapy include progressive muscular relaxation (which can be learned from tapes if no live therapist is available) and hypnosis.

COGNITIVE THERAPY (Moorey and Greer 1989)

First developed for treating depression and anxiety in physically healthy people, cognitive therapy is now applied by psychologists, psychiatrists and other mental health professionals to a much wider range of disorders. Whilst being a separate technique in its own right, cognitive therapy provides something of a middle ground between the psychodynamic and the behavioural schools already described.

According to cognitive theory, emotional problems arise and/or continue because of maladaptive beliefs and thinking patterns. The emotional threat of cancer depends on a patient's 'cognitive schema' derived from individual past experience. Some of the resulting beliefs may be distorted. An elderly man, whose father died a horrid death from cancer many years before modern pain-relief techniques became available, may hold the belief 'you always die in agony with cancer'. A young woman with breast cancer, whose self-esteem is closely bound up with her physical appearance, may hold the belief 'no man wants a woman with only one breast'. Both are black-and-white statements, understandable in the light of these patients' personalities and past experience, but neither accurate nor helpful in relation to their present plight.

In therapy, patients are encouraged to identify their 'automatic negative thoughts', reconsider these more logically, and experiment with alternative viewpoints and behaviours which give them a greater sense of control over the situation. Steven Greer and Stirling Moorey and their colleagues at the Royal Marsden Hospital have shown cognitive therapy to be useful in the management of depression and anxiety following the diagnosis of cancer.

Specific techniques include:

- Identify, record and eventually challenge negative automatic thoughts.
- Rehearse impending stressful events and ways of handling these, through imagination and role play.
- Plan and carry out practical activities which instil a sense of mastery, control and pleasure.
- Express feelings openly to one's partner.
- Raise self-esteem by identifying and fostering personal strengths.

Therapy focuses on current problems as identified by the patient; denial, if present, need not be challenged. The treatment contract for formal therapy might be between six and twelve weekly sessions, each lasting one hour. Progress between sessions is monitored through use of a diary kept by the patient. The spouse or partner may be included. Cognitive therapy is often combined with practical behavioural methods, and relaxation training.

Like other formal psychotherapies, cognitive therapy is unsuitable as a main treatment for patients with major psychiatric illness or organic brain syndromes; and it is more applicable for patients with early cancers than advanced ones. Its use in advanced disease would often seem inappropriate, because patients' fear and pessimism are often amply justified by their real situation. A selective commonsense application of the cognitive approach, however, sometimes does help in such cases.

Peter, aged 62, knew that his bowel cancer had spread to his liver and he had only weeks or months to live, although his current physical condition remained reasonably good. He took the view 'let's get it over as quick as we can' and stated that he would certainly want euthanasia if this were available. Having had to give up the job which was important to him, and abandon a longterm plan for renovating a French farmhouse for his retirement, he gave up all other activities as well, on the grounds that there was no point in doing anything but wait for death. In cognitive terms he could be said to be using 'all or none reasoning' and 'catastrophising'.

continued

continued

After discussion of his attitudes, and a review of the way he was spending his day, he began to acknowledge that he was taking a black-and-white view of things and that certain aspects of his life might yet be worthwhile after all. He agreed to resume some of the activities which had given him pleasure in the past—for example visiting local beauty spots, even though he now had to travel as a passenger in a car rather than on his own bicycle—and his daily diary of mood and activities showed that, once he had overcome his inertia in getting started, such outings were indeed followed by improvement in his mood. He also took on a more active role in decisions about his treatment; having previously said merely 'let the hospital decide' when offered some palliative chemotherapy, he drew up a written list of its likely pros and cons before making a positive decision not to proceed. The improvement in Peter's mood was sustained as he gradually became weaker, and though his range of activities became more limited, he continued to take pleasure in them.

PATIENT SUPPORT GROUPS (Mastrovito, Moynihan and Parsonnet 1989)

Group meetings for patients with cancer provide a forum for sharing feelings, exchanging practical information, and giving and receiving psychological support. They differ in a number of ways from the kind of formal therapy groups used in psychiatric settings. Most patients attending a cancer support group do not have severe emotional problems—for those who do, individual therapy is often better. A personal experience of running a support group in a hospice day centre for patients with advanced cancer will be described here. Many other models could be used, the choice depending both on the patient population concerned and the background of the group leader(s).

Many people find the idea of 'group therapy' alarming and off-putting. In order to give potential members some idea of the purpose and format of our group, a one-page hand-out was prepared. This outlined the kind of problems which many cancer patients experience—anxiety about the future, coping with loss of independence, feeling isolated from other people—and stated the group's aim of providing a comfortable, friendly setting where such problems, and ways of coping with them, could be shared. The practical organisation was described and the three ground rules—confidentiality, punctuality and no-smoking—set out.

Two staff members came to each meeting. Although ideally these would have been the same people each time, practical considerations dictated that in order to keep the group going continuously over a long period, we needed a larger rota. A social worker, an occupational therapist, and several Macmillan nurses took part besides myself. The number of patients attending varied between three and eight. Regular attendance was encouraged but could not be enforced, because failing health or other hospital appointments often intervened.

Meetings took place once a week and lasted one hour. The group leader welcomed any new members, and everyone present introduced themselves, using first names only. Fifty minutes of discussion followed, and then a ten-minute relaxation exercise. It was necessary for the leaders to spend time each week to make sure the practical organisation—transport arrangements, supplying drinks and tissues—worked smoothly. We chose to have free-ranging conversation on whatever topics patients raised that day. Frequent themes included:

- *Family relationships*: most patients considered their relatives an important source of support, yet might find it difficult to talk with them about the illness. Some felt their spouses or children were avoiding the situation, for example the woman whose husband resisted her efforts to teach him to cook. Many relatives seemed unable to find the right balance between overprotecting the patient, and expecting him or her to cope as before. Men who had been forced to give up work felt diminished by their inability to support their families. Patients often expressed guilt about being ill when a family holiday had been planned or when their children were preparing for exams. We tried to reassure patients that their relatives still valued them although their practical role was curtailed.
- *Communication with doctors and nurses*: patients expressed a clear wish for frank and full communication. They approved of being allowed to see their casenotes and X-rays, and if the result of a test was unfavourable they preferred to be told as much directly. At the same time, some showed reluctance to ask

questions or 'bother the doctor', and tended to seek paternalistic guidance and clearcut answers to complex clinical dilemmas.

- *Practical activities*: giving up driving the car was often seen as the ultimate loss of independence, although one or two members could see advantages such as saving hassle and money. The need for flexibility and compromise regarding their lifestyle was hard for some to accept, though a few had considered less demanding sorts of work or had taken up new hobbies such as model-boat making. Exchanging tips about the aids available—ranging from kitchen gadgets to concessionary theatre tickets—was evidently helpful.

- *Social interactions*: patients often criticised other people's reactions to their illness. Some complained that friends ignored them; others claimed that strangers stared, or acquaintances came to visit out of morbid curiosity. Offering practical help, without taking over completely, was usually welcomed. Fear of vomiting or fits in public places such as supermarkets, combined with problems of wheelchair access, added to restrictions on activity.

- *Death and dying*: many members spoke of these issues with matter-of-fact directness, for example describing their own funeral plans. From time to time, inevitably, group members actually did die; perhaps having attended a group meeting just a few days before. The other members consistently made it clear that they wanted to know of such events, rather than be left wondering about somebody who had 'disappeared' and not liking to ask why, so the deaths were always acknowledged. The degree of discussion about them, however, varied considerably. With occasional striking exceptions, death and dying did not take up a large part of group time. The open group structure, with its constantly changing membership, probably weighed against too much personal disclosure on these sensitive issues. Also, most members did not seem to want too serious a group culture, preferring the meetings to have a friendly and positive atmosphere.

A practical disadvantage of the deaths was continual depletion of group attendance. If numbers and morale were in danger of sagging too far, we might arrange a month's planned break while recruiting some new members.

Most patients, even shy ones who said very little, seemed to find the group helpful and many examples of mutual support were apparent. We were not aware of any major problems although there were several minor ones. Brain tumour patients, and others with organic impairments, often had trouble in expressing themselves with regard to abstract psychological concepts. With such patients present, the therapists had to play a fairly active role to maintain a meaningful discussion rather than letting long silences or excess superficial chatter ('Did you watch the match last night?') take over. Black humour once threatened to get out of hand; one member told a story about a guinea-pig being sucked into a vacuum cleaner, and this provoked a round of similar gruesome anecdotes from the others, no doubt representing defences against material of a more personal kind.

Just one type of group has been described here. Many others are possible: a self-help group run outside hospital premises by patients themselves, or structured educational meetings based on talks from visiting experts. Whatever its format, a group involving patient-to-patient interaction offers something quite distinct from professional counselling or psychotherapy.

PSYCHOTROPIC DRUGS (Massie and Lesko 1989)

Psychotropic drugs fall into three main groups: *antidepressants*, *hypnotics and anxiolytics* (sedatives) and *neuroleptics*. Psychotropic drugs have many uses in oncology, for example in the management of organic brain syndromes, and the control of nausea and pain. This section is concerned mainly with the drug treatment of depression and anxiety (mood disorders).

When should Drug Treatment be Considered?

The differences between natural worry and clinical anxiety, and between natural sadness and clinical depression, have already been discussed. Most cancer patients go through phases of worry and sadness during their illness, but these may be part of an adjustment process for which psychotropic drugs are neither appropriate nor effective. These normal reactions merge into the more severe and prolonged forms of anxiety and depression, for which drug treatment may well be helpful. In general, the more severe and acute the mood disorder, the better its response to psychotropic drugs.

Mood disorder secondary to organic factors such as cerebral metastases or hypercalcaemia may also be helped by drugs, although the starting dose should be lower than usual because of the risk of confusion. Obviously, the underlying medical condition should be treated directly if that is possible.

Why Psychotropic Drugs are Under-used

In most cancer treatment settings, psychotropic drugs—especially antidepressants—are prescribed only for a minority of the patients who might benefit. Several factors contribute to under-prescribing.

Firstly, mood disorders are often unrecognised. Most patients do not raise emotional problems unless asked, and staff very often fail to ask because they are short of time and/or would be unsure how to deal with any problems revealed.

Secondly, many oncologists are unfamiliar with psychotropic drugs, and are concerned about possible adverse effects in frail patients who may be taking large amounts of medication already.

Thirdly, several misunderstandings regarding psychotropic drugs discourage their use. There is a widespread but illogical belief that mood disorders in cancer patients do not merit drug treatment, because these patients have such obvious reason to feel depressed and anxious. In reality, it is better to decide the need for treatment on the basis of the symptom pattern of the mood disorder, rather than its (presumed) cause. Another mistaken belief is that drugs are incompatible with psychological treatments. Some people equate taking psychotropic drugs with moral weakness, and assume that counselling must be better. The evidence, however, shows that a combination of antidepressant drugs and psychological treatments works better than either one alone. Lastly, there are concerns about addiction and dependence, which may be valid in relation to the longterm use of benzodiazepines, but seldom for antidepressants.

Antidepressant Drugs

These are the best drugs to choose for patients with a sustained mood disorder, whether depression or anxiety predominates. In ordinary psychiatric practice, about 70% of depressed patients respond well to antidepressants, which are also effective for anxiety states and panic disorder. The response rate in patients with serious physical disorders such as cancer appears, perhaps surprisingly, to be equally high but there have been few controlled trials. Antidepressants may help relieve insomnia, pain, and loss of appetite, whether these symptoms arise from depression or from cancer.

Tricyclic antidepressants such as *amitriptyline, imipramine* and *dothiepin* are well-established as standard therapy for depressive illness. They modify cerebral monoamine neurotransmitter systems involving 5-hydroxytryptamine (5-HT, serotonin) and/or noradrenaline (NA).

Tricyclics have many potential adverse effects, mostly due to their anticholinergic properties. Dry mouth, constipation, dizziness due to postural hypotension, blurred vision, and sweating may occur. Drowsiness is sometimes a problem, but because most depressed patients suffer from insomnia, this can often be turned to advantage by giving the total dose at bedtime. Weight gain, though unwelcome for most depressives in the general population, may be an advantage for those with cancer. Confusion may develop if antidepressants are given to patients with metabolic disturbances or organic brain disease, and caution is required in the presence of cardiovascular disease, glaucoma, prostatic enlargement or liver failure. Unwanted effects are usually most prominent in the first few days of treatment, whereas the benefits may take several weeks to become evident. Overdose may cause death through respiratory depression, cardiac arrhythmia or status epilepticus. Though this long list of potential problems may sound alarming, most patients with moderate or severe depression tolerate the tricyclics well.

More recently-developed antidepressant drugs, such as *mianserin* and *lofepramine,* are similar in efficacy to the older tricyclics but often better tolerated, and are safer in overdose. *Specific serotonin reuptake inhibitors (SSRIs),* namely *fluoxetine, fluvoxamine, paroxetine* and *sertraline* are currently popular;

nausea, often transient, is their main unwanted effect. All these drugs are more expensive than the older tricyclics.

Monoamine oxidase inhibitors (MAOIs) such as *phenelzine, isocarboxazid* and *tranylcypromine* are sometimes highly effective for patients who have failed to respond to other antidepressants. However, they may be dangerous if mixed with certain other drugs and foodstuffs. Because of their drug interactions, MAOIs are not the ideal choice for cancer patients undergoing active medical or surgical treatment, but might be considered for those in physical remission. A new variant of this group called *RIMAs* (reversible inhibitors of monoamine oxidase A), less prone to drug interactions, has just been introduced; *moclobemide* is the first example.

Lithium and *carbamazepine* are used mainly as longterm mood stabilisers for patients who suffer repeated episodes of depression or manic-depression.

This list of antidepressant drugs is not complete; the British National Formulary lists around 30 different compounds. Sometimes there are logical reasons for selecting a particular one, for example amitriptyline would be a good choice for an agitated patient who could not sleep, but a bad choice for a patient with cardiac arrhythmia. In many clinical situations, however, there is little to choose between one antidepressant and another.

Dose and duration of therapy: it is most important to give an adequate dose and persevere for sufficient time. Tricyclics such as amitriptyline and imipramine have a wide therapeutic dose range; anything from 10 to 250 mg daily, usually between 75 and 150 mg. The dose should be built up over a period of days or weeks to the maximum level the individual can tolerate. The newer drugs are simpler to use in this respect; for example the standard dose of both fluoxetine and paroxetine is 20 mg daily and there is little point in giving more. Many patients begin to improve within a week or two of starting antidepressant treatment, but others take four to six weeks to respond. Patients must be warned of this delay, otherwise they may give up the drug after the first few days.

If the antidepressant proves successful, another common mistake is stopping it too soon. Many patients are keen to do without drugs as soon as they feel better. However, relapse is much less likely if medication is continued for about six months before being gradually tapered off.

Electroconvulsive therapy (ECT) is not a drug, but may be mentioned here as a rapid and effective treatment for severe depression. It tends to be reserved for patients who are suicidal, or refusing food and drink. ECT involves the passage of a small electric current across one or both temples. This is not so frightening as it sounds, because the patient is given a short-acting general anaesthetic plus a muscle relaxant beforehand. Observers will see a slight twitching, of which the patient is unaware. The procedure is repeated every few days until the depression is better; at least six treatments are usually required. Some patients experience headache and confusion for a few hours after treatment, and may suffer a disturbance of recent memory lasting several weeks. Permanent memory damage is not recorded.

ECT is very occasionally indicated for depressed cancer patients. Although it is a safe treatment which can be successfully given to the elderly and frail, caution is required for patients with cardiac or respiratory disease who are at risk of anaesthetic complications; those with bony metastases who are at risk of pathological fracture; and those with raised intracranial pressure. The decision to prescribe ECT for a medically sick depressed patient should be made only by an experienced psychiatrist, working in collaboration with an experienced anaesthetist. Except in extremely rare circumstances, a course of ECT requires informed consent from the patient.

Anxiolytics and Hypnotics

These drugs are useful for the short-term or episodic treatment of anxiety or insomnia. For more sustained mood disorders, even if the symptoms suggest anxiety rather than depression, the antidepressant drugs described above are better. This is because anxiolytics taken continuously for more than two or three weeks tend to lose their therapeutic effect and/or create dependence.

Anxiolytics are best reserved for times of crisis. Patients being investigated for the initial symptoms of cancer or for a suspected recurrence, and relatives who are newly bereaved, may become acutely distressed and a short course of anxiolytics or hypnotics (for those who want this) will help tide them over the worst.

Some purists would argue on principle against the use of drugs at such times of adjustment and transition. This view seems unduly harsh. Of course it is bad practice to hand out drugs automatically, to use them as a substitute for talking through the crisis, or to allow that crisis to become a starting-point for longterm drug use.

Anxiolytics are also useful in situation-specific anxiety. Patients who feel highly threatened by injections, X-rays or even clinic visits may benefit from a single dose beforehand—or just from knowing they have a tablet in their pocket.

Benzodiazepines are the most widely used anxiolytics today, although since the risk of dependence was recognised and publicised in the 1980s, some doctors and patients are reluctant to use them at all. This is a pity, because they are effective and safe for short-term use. They have few side-effects, and are safe in overdose. A few patients, however, develop a 'paradoxical' reaction of aggression and disinhibition.

Benzodiazepines differ in their potency and duration of action. Some are marketed as daytime anxiolytics, others as bedtime hypnotics. Examples include *diazepam* (long-acting anxiolytic), *lorazepam* (short-acting anxiolytic), and *temazepam* (hypnotic).

Patients who are dependent on benzodiazepines have great difficulty in coming off their medication, even if it does not seem to be helping them much, and abrupt withdrawal may cause intense anxiety, nausea, trembling and even fits. Partly because of this, longterm prescription is now frowned upon, and many family doctors have made great efforts to wean benzodiazepine users off their drugs. For patients with cancer, a somewhat different attitude may be required. For someone recently diagnosed with life-threatening illness, for example, it is probably not timely to try to come off benzodiazepines; and for someone with only limited life expectancy, there may be no point in worrying about dependence, or attempting withdrawal for those who are dependent already.

Beta-blockers such as *propranolol* are useful for patients whose anxiety takes the form of physical symptoms such as tremor, palpitations or muscle tension. *Neuroleptics* such as *haloperidol* are effective in calming acute disturbance in the physically ill.

Barbiturates are effective anxiolytics, seldom prescribed nowadays because of their potential for dependence, and toxicity in overdose, but occasionally used when other drugs have failed.

The Place of Psychotropic Drugs in Cancer Patient Care

Psychotropic drugs, like any other treatment, should be prescribed only by a doctor with knowledge and experience of their use. This doctor need not be a psychiatrist. Many general practitioners (GPs) are skilled in the use of these drugs, and a GP who knows the patient's past history may be the most suitable person to decide about prescribing them. In the hospital, cancer specialists who learn about two or three of the commonly-used psychotropics will be able to prescribe successfully for many of their patients. Psychiatric advice will be required if the case is unusually complex, if the advisability of using drugs at all is in doubt, or if the first-line drugs fail to work.

Drugs have a central role in managing the more severe emotional disorders found among cancer patients—but on their own are not enough. Drugs should never be used as a quick substitute for listening to patients and building up a therapeutic relationship. Specialised treatments in psycho-oncology, whether by psychotherapy or drugs, only work well in a setting where the skilled treatment of the cancer itself is combined with good communication, good staff–patient relationships, and an understanding acceptance of emotional distress.

FURTHER READING

Breitbart W, Holland JC (eds) (1993) *Psychiatric Aspects of Symptom Management in Cancer Patients.* Washington: American Psychiatric Press

Brown D, Pedder J (1991) *Introduction to Psychotherapy.* London: Routledge

Davis H, Fallowfield L (eds) (1991) *Counselling and Communication in Health Care.* Chichester: Wiley

Massie MJ, Lesko LM. Psychopharmacological management. In Holland JC, Rowland JH (eds) (1989) *Handbook of Psychooncology.* Oxford University Press: New York

Mastrovito R. Behavioural techniques: progressive relaxation and self-regulatory therapies. In Holland JC, Rowland JH (eds) (1989) *Handbook of Psychooncology* . Oxford University Press: New York

Mastrovito R, Moynihan RT, Parsonnet L. Self-help and mutual support programmes. In Holland JC, Rowland JH (eds) (1989) *Handbook of Psychooncology* . Oxford University Press: New York

Moorey S, Greer S (1989) *Psychological Therapy for Patients with Cancer*. Oxford: Heinemann

Watson M (1983) Psychosocial intervention with cancer patients: a review. *Psychological Medicine 13* 839–46

Watson M (ed) (1991) *Cancer Patient Care: Psychosocial Treatment Methods*. Cambridge: BPS Books

Psychometric Measurement Scales

Anxiety and depression:
Zigmond AS, Snaith RP (1983) The Hospital Anxiety and Depression (HAD) Scale. *Acta Psychiatrica Scandinavica* 67 361–370

Attitude to cancer:
Watson M, Greer S, Young J, Inayat Q, Burgess C, Robertson B (1988) Development of a questionnaire measure of adjustment to cancer: the MAC Scale. *Psychological Medicine* 18 203–209

Quality of life:
de Haes JCJM, van Knippenberg FCE, Neijt JP (1990) Measuring psychological and physical distress in cancer patients: structure and application of the Rotterdam Symptom Checklist. *British Journal of Cancer* 62 1034–8

Cognitive impairment:
Folstein MF, Folstein SE, McHugh PR (1975) Mini-mental state: a practical method of grading the cognitive state of patients for the clinician. *Journal of Psychiatric Research* 12 189–98

These are only a few examples of the many scales available. The book edited by Chris Thompson (1989) *The Instruments of Psychiatric Research*, published by Wiley, Chichester, gives many others. For copyright reasons, the scales themselves cannot be reproduced here.

Addresses

BACUP (British Association of Cancer United Patients)
3 Bath Place
Rivington St
London
EC2A 3JR
Tel: 071 613 2121; Freeline from outside London 0800 181199

Cancer Link
17 Britannia St
London
WCX 9JN
Tel: 071 833 2451

Both organisations offer factual information and emotional support to people affected by cancer.

CRUSE—Bereavement Care
126 Sheen Rd
Richmond
Surrey
TW9 1UR
Tel: 081 940 4818; helpline 081 332 7227

Voluntary organisation offering individual and group support to bereaved people. Branches throughout the country.

BPOG (British Psychosocial Oncology Group)
Membership Secretary
Cancer support and information
Mount Vernon Hospital
Northwood
Middlesex
HA6 2RN
Tel: 0895 278014

A society for healthcare professionals interested in clinical or research aspects of psychosocial oncology. Annual conference, journal (*Psycho-oncology*) and newsletter.

GLOSSARY

Adenocarcinoma: a carcinoma originating from glandular tissue

Adjuvant treatment: additional treatment by radiotherapy and/or chemotherapy given to destroy any residual cancer cells left behind after surgery

Affect: mood

Akathisia: restlessness of mind and body caused by malfunction of the extrapyramidal system; a side-effect of neuroleptic drugs

Amitriptyline: an antidepressant drug of the tricyclic group

Androgen: male sex hormone

Axillary lymph nodes: the lymph nodes under the armpit which are the usual first site for metastasis of breast cancer

Benign: non-malignant, non-cancerous

Benzodiazepines: a group of anxiolytic and hypnotic drugs, also called minor tranquillisers

Biopsy: removal of a small portion of tissue for histological examination

Bone scan: a special X-ray which may be used to detect metastases of cancer in bones

Carcinogenic: capable of causing or contributing to cancer

Carcinoma: a common type of cancer, arising from epithelial tissue

Cell: the smallest unit in the body which is capable of independent function. Visible under a microscope

Cerebral: relating to the brain

Cervix (adj. cervical): neck of the womb

Chemotherapy: drug treatment, esp. cytotoxic drugs

Chlorpromazine: a neuroleptic drug

Clinical depression: depressive illness

Cognitive: concerned with intellectual functions such as perception, thought, memory, reasoning

Cognitive therapy: a form of psychotherapy which uses reasoning processes to address emotional problems

Colostomy: surgical formation of an opening from the colon (large bowel) onto the body surface. Sometimes necessary for patients with cancer of the rectum or colon

Conversion: the manifestation of repressed emotion in the form of bodily symptoms (conversion hysteria)

Cortisone: a steroid hormone produced in the adrenal gland

Counselling: listening to problems and offering information and advice

CT (or CAT): computed axial tomography, a type of X-ray scan which can be used to visualise cancer in various body parts

Delirium: clouding of consciousness often accompanied by delusions and hallucinations, due to acute organic brain disease

Delusion: a false belief, not in keeping with the beliefs of the subject's social group, which persists despite evidence against it

Dementia: chronic, usually irreversible, impairment of cognitive function due to organic brain disease

Denial: unconsciously ignoring some threatening aspect of reality in order to protect the ego against anxiety

Depression:
1. a mood state of sadness, a normal reaction to loss
2. depressive illness (clinical depression)

Dexamethasone: a steroid drug

Displacement: the transfer of emotion from the person or object which caused it towards a different and more acceptable target

ECT: electroconvulsive therapy, a treatment for severe depressive illness

Ego: the conscious part of the mind which deals with everyday reality. A theoretical concept associated with Sigmund Freud

Endogenous depression: depressive illness which cannot be explained by stressful life circumstances

Euphoria: exaggerated elation

Fluoxetine: an antidepressant drug
Fluvoxamine: an antidepressant drug

Genetic: inherited

Hallucination: a false perception arising in the absence of an appropriate external stimulus. Auditory hallucinations ('hearing voices') are characteristic of psychiatric illness; visual hallucinations ('seeing things') are characteristic of organic brain syndromes

Haloperidol: a neuroleptic drug

Histology: study of tissue under a microscope. Used to confirm a diagnosis of cancer and determine the cell type

Hodgkin's disease: a type of lymphoma

Hormone: a chemical, produced by an endocrine gland, which circulates in the blood and exerts effects on other parts of the body

Hypercalcaemia: raised blood calcium. May occur as a complication of cancer

Hypochondriasis: excessive concern about physical health

Hysterectomy: removal of the womb

Identification: assumption of the characteristics of another person, usually someone admired by, or similar to, oneself

Illusion: a perceptual distortion whereby a stimulus is misinterpreted

Imipramine: an antidepressant drug

Immune system: bodily defences against disease. Includes antibodies and lymphocytes

Intellectualisation: explaining emotional issues in logical, rational terms

Laryngectomy: removal of the larynx (voice box)

Latent period: the time during which cancer is growing in the body but has not yet given rise to clinical symptoms

Leukaemia: a type of cancer arising in the bone marrow and involving overproduction of white cells in the blood

Lumpectomy: surgical removal of a cancer without removing the whole organ in which it has arisen. Mostly applied to breast cancer

Lymph nodes: bean-shaped masses of tissue, found in various parts of the body, containing lymphocytes—cells which protect against infection and other diseases

Lymphoma: a type of cancer arising in lymph nodes or lymphoid tissue

Mania: a psychiatric illness characterised by elation of mood and overactivity

MAOIs: monoamine oxidase inhibitors, a group of antidepressant drugs

Mastectomy: removal of a breast

Melanoma: a form of skin cancer, often developing from a mole

Metabolic disturbance: derangement of body chemistry

Metastases: secondary deposits of cancer in parts of the body other than the organ of origin

Mianserin: an antidepressant drug

Moclobemide: an antidepressant drug

Mood disorders (affective disorders): a group of psychiatric illnesses including depression, anxiety and mania

MRI: magnetic resonance imaging, a type of X-ray scan which can be used to visualise cancer in various body parts

Myeloma: a cancer originating from B-lymphocytes, usually involving bone marrow, and producing abnormal immunoglobulins in the blood

Neoplasm: 'new growth', often used as another term for cancer

Neuroleptics: antipsychotic drugs, major tranquillisers

Oestrogen: female sex hormone

Organic brain syndromes: conditions caused by physical disease of the brain itself, or by chemical disturbances (resulting from disease of other organs, or from drugs) which disturb brain function

Palliative treatment: treatment to relieve symptoms when the underlying disease cannot be cured

Pancreas: an abdominal organ which produces insulin, also certain enzymes for digestion of food

Paranoid: suspicious, fearful of persecution

Paraplegia: paralysis of the lower part of the body

Paroxetine: an antidepressant drug

Personality: habitual behavioural and mental traits, characteristic of the individual concerned

Phobia: excessive fear of a specific object or situation

Prednisolone: a steroid drug

Primary site: the place in the body where a cancer originally developed

Projection: attributing one's own, usually unacceptable, feelings to other people

Prospective study: a research design in which subjects are followed up to observe relationships between their original characteristics and what happens to them later (cf. retrospective)

Prosthesis: an artificial substitute for a missing body part

Psychosomatic: physiological dysfunction secondary to mental factors

Psychotherapy: treatment through the exchange of words and feelings within a professional relationship

Radical treatment: intensive treatment aimed to cure

Rationalisation: unconsciously finding a logical reason for thoughts or beliefs which are really determined by emotions of an unacknowledged or unacceptable kind

Regression: literally 'moving backwards'. Used:
1. in cancer medicine to mean shrinking of a tumour, usually after successful treatment
2. in psychiatry to mean reverting back to feelings or behaviour appropriate to an earlier stage of life

Repression: an unconscious 'mental mechanism' in which something threatening or unacceptable is forgotten or ignored

Retrospective study: a research design in which patients who already have the condition of interest are questioned about their past, to seek possible causes. A comparison group of people without the condition is usually included (cf. prospective)

Sarcoma: a rare type of cancer arising from connective tissue

Sertraline: an antidepressant drug

Somatic: bodily, physical

Somatisation: expression of unacknowledged emotional distress in the guise of physical complaints

Squamous cell carcinoma: a cancer originating from a type of epithelial cell

Steroid: a group of chemicals, including naturally-produced hormones from the adrenal gland and synthesised drugs, with widespread physiological effects. They are sometimes useful in cancer treatment

Sublimation: redirection of frustrated desires into socially acceptable channels

Suppression: deliberately excluding something unpleasant from one's thoughts

Systemic: affecting the body as a whole

Tamoxifen: a drug, an oestrogen receptor antagonist, used in treatment of breast cancer

Tissue: part of the body consisting of a large number of cells having a similar structure and function

Transference: emotions which the subject experienced towards someone in the past are projected onto another person. Often used in the context of a patient's feelings towards a psychotherapist. 'Countertransference' is the reverse, the therapist's feelings towards the patient

Tumour: an abnormal mass of tissue caused by excess growth of cells. May be cancerous (malignant) or benign (non-malignant)

Index

Index compiled by Campbell Purton and Jennifer Barraclough